# The Art of Surgical Technique

# The Art of Surgical Technique

## Milton T. Edgerton, M.D., F.A.C.S.

Professor and Chairman
Department of Plastic and Maxillofacial Surgery
The University of Virginia Medical Center
Charlottesville, Virginia

Illustrated by

## Florence J. Kabir, M.F.A.

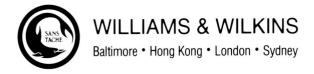

WILLIAMS & WILKINS
Baltimore • Hong Kong • London • Sydney

*Editor:* Kimberly Kist
*Associate Editor:* Victoria M. Vaughn
*Production and Manufacturing:* Bermedica Production

In most of the text, the pronoun "he" is used to refer to the surgeon or surgical assistant and the pronoun "she" refers to the nurse. This is done for linguistic simplicity and grammatical convenience. It is not intended to be discriminatory. The rapid increase in the number of women entering the surgical profession may soon change our traditional notion of surgery as a profession for men.

Copyright © 1988
Williams & Wilkins
428 East Preston Street
Baltimore, MD 21202, USA

Accurate indications, adverse reactions, and dosage schedules for drugs are provided in this book, but it is possible that they may change. The reader is urged to review the package information data of the manufacturers of the medications mentioned.

Printed in the United States of America

**Library of Congress Cataloging-in-Publication Data**

Edgerton, Milton T., 1921-
    The art of surgical technique.

    Includes bibliographies and index.
    1. Surgery, Operative. I. Title. [DNLM: 1. Surgery,
Operative. WO 500 E23a]
RD32.E34   1988       617'.91       87-25446
ISBN 0-683-02749-2 (paperback)
ISBN 0-683-02750-6 (case)

Composed by Waldman Graphics, Inc.                88 89 90 91
                                      1 2 3 4 5 6 7 8 9 10

*To Patricia*

*with deepest appreciation for all of her encouragement, loyalty, humor, and good sense. A special note of thanks is indicated for her tolerance during those early years in which her kitchen towels were being sutured together with all manner of materials, stitches, and knots.*

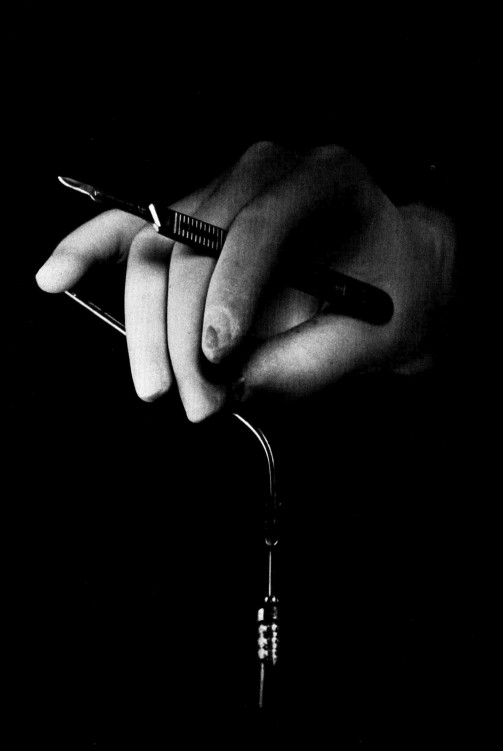

# Foreword

Writing the foreword for this book by Dr. Milton Edgerton gives me great personal pleasure and satisfaction. I first met him during World War II when he joined our busy team caring for the wounded at Valley Forge General Hospital in Pennsylvania. He was one of that outstanding group of young surgeons who established such an enviable record of patient care both during the war and in the years since. Following the subsequent careers of each of these surgeons has been impressive. Milton Edgerton has certainly lived up to the promise evident in those early years.

In compiling this treatise on surgical technique based on his many hours in the operating room and on his numerous original contributions to the art, the author has rendered an important service to all surgeons without regard to specialty. To the mature surgeon, the teaching of the minutiae of surgical technique can become tedious, with the lingering hope that trainees may have a natural sixth sense or an inherent prompt grasp without repeated admonitions. Thus not only to trainees but to surgeons of all ages, this book will be a ready source of instructive information.

The author has had the good fortune of finding a skilled medical artist in the person of Ms. Florence Kabir, a gifted illustrator and photographer whose drawings are an essential part of the book. She has succeeded in accurately picturing the step-by-step sequences from the simple maneuver of tying a square knot to the most highly complex procedure. Descriptive explanations in the text serve to clarify the details of each step.

In the operating room the responsibilities of the members of the surgical team, especially those of the first assistant, are outlined. He must anticipate each step in the operation to ensure the smooth running of the procedure. One is reminded of the often-quoted adage that, a good first assistant can make a clumsy surgeon look great, but a poor first assistant can make a competent surgeon look bad. A good assistant can be expected to develop into a skillful senior surgeon.

Thoughtful etiquette in the operating room is part of proper surgical technique. The author emphasizes that quiet is essential even in a teaching setting whether the patient is awake or under general anesthesia. Implied is talking in a low voice, the use of hand signals in calling for instruments, and suppressed noise from necessary operating room equipment.

The gentle handling of all tissues is addressed in each chapter, with suggestions about the careful placement of retractors, with moist gauze padding if possible, the use of skin hooks (single or multiple), and, finally, blunt dissection with that most useful of all instruments, the finger!

All surgeons with wide experience are fully aware of the many surgical pitfalls and promptly learn to avoid them. The author has seen his share and warns his readers to be alert lest they make the same mistakes. In enumerating several obvious ones, he furnishes advice to the novice but older surgeons will also find his observations of value.

That the author is left-handed is apparent judging from the several comments in the text about left-handed scissors vs right-handed scissors, and the dilemma of on which side of the table the left-handed surgeon should stand in this right-handed world. Also quite apparent is his remarkable self-taught ambidexterity which he recognizes as a necessity in performing a goodly number of plastic surgical procedures.

Finally, Dr. Edgerton writes gratefully about the frequent expressions of appreciation from former residents thanking him for techniques learned during the training years which have proven of continuing value. These are among the many rewards of having a part in the passing on of knowledge whether by example, by word of mouth, or by publishing a book on *The Art of Surgical Technique*.

Bradford Cannon, M.D.
Clinical Professor of Surgery Emeritus
Harvard Medical School;
Senior Surgeon
Massachusetts General Hospital
Boston, Massachusetts

# Foreword

Plastic surgeons are by necessity obsessive about the delicate and appropriate handling of tissues. For centuries their work was largely confined to the skin where any imperfections in healing were at once obvious. Fortunately, even today when the scope of plastic surgery has become so extensive and operations of great magnitude are within the realm of plastic surgery its devotees retain the gentleness and precision that have ever been their hallmarks. It is entirely proper therefore, that a book on *The Art of Surgical Technique* should have been written by a plastic surgeon.

Dr. Edgerton has years of experience in the broadest realms of plastic surgery and his extensive laboratory investigations might have led one to expect that he would turn at this point in his career to a massive and sophisticated tome for the experts in his field. What a pleasure and what a delight it is to find that this master surgeon has chosen to provide in this elegant little book the simplest and most basic description of techniques, the appropriate utilization of which are a joy to behold and a blessing to the patients whose tissues are thus elegantly manipulated. Although some of the illustrations deal with examples taken from operations that are recognizedly those of plastic surgery, the principles and details are those that apply to all surgery. In this day of antibiotics, complicated anesthesia techniques, and recovery room and ICU resuscitation technology, many of us have had a feeling that too little stress has been laid upon the techniques of elegant and precise surgery. Our 1,500 page—and more—surgical texts do not tell us how to use a knife, how to use a scissors, how to use forceps and which ones to use; how to apply hemostats, how to ligate or transfix vessels, how to place sutures or how to cut them; Dr. Edgerton's book does. Where else would you find on page after page, an analysis of what the first assistant should be doing, how he should be doing it, and why? Where else will you find mention of the left-handed surgeon, his problems, and the problems of the assistant opposite him (of course Dr. Edgerton is left-handed, as he says some 25% of plastic surgeons turn out to be)? Where else will you find a discussion of knot tying, the suture materials, the needles, the methods of putting needles through the tissue and the methods of drawing them out, and all of this in simple, lucid language with elegant and simple illustrations? Where else will you find descriptions and illustrations of the hand signals conventionally used in operating rooms?

This charming book is one that medical students interested in surgery would do well to read and reread, and that surgical residents in their first years, when they are beginning to operate, should master. Not many of their teachers have the patience or the interest or have been analytical enough to transmit the information Dr. Edgerton provides.

Mark M. Ravitch, M.D.
Professor of Surgery
University of Pittsburgh;
Surgeon-in-Chief, Emeritus
The Montefiore Hospital
Pittsburgh, Pennsylvania

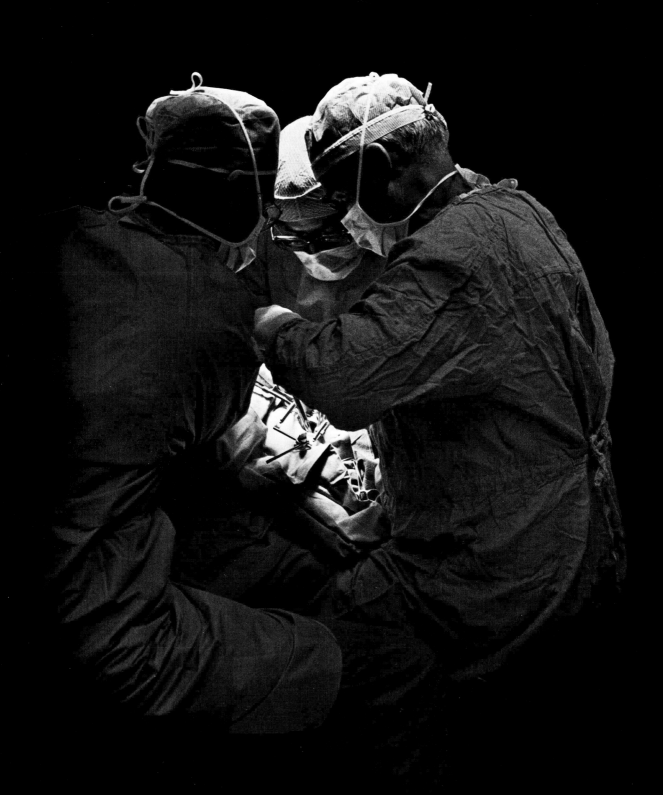

# Preface

*Chyrurgerie is an art, which teacheth the way by reason, how by the operation of the hand we may cure, prevent and mitigate diseases, which accidentally happen upon us.*

*Ambroise Paré, 1582*

I have spent over forty thousand hours at the operating table alongside young men and women as they acquired basic surgical techniques and skills. To some, the handling of tools and tissues comes easily—almost without their conscious realization. Others must laboriously learn the many subtle ways that surgeons use their hands to support, expose, remove, manipulate, and repair the tissues of the human body. These movements must be efficient, time-saving, and gentle enough to avoid undue damage to living cells. They require the almost unconscious integration of rather complex movements of both hands.

The hands of the principal surgeon are usually engaged in accomplishing the primary objectives of the operation. The hands of the assistant surgeons must expedite that surgeon's work. This interplay of cooperating hands can produce a flowing and beautiful pattern of teamwork—or, if done badly, it can result in a rough, halting, awkward, and time-consuming exercise. This book is an effort to record many of the pointers used by the author to help young surgeons to use their hands and tools in ways that will encourage tissue to heal well. I have found that these techniques make the long hours spent in the operating room a more pleasurable experience. They are methods and movements that should be of value to general surgeons, plastic surgeons, orthopedic surgeons, urologists, neurosurgeons, gynecologists, thoracic surgeons, pediatric surgeons, oral surgeons, otolaryngologists, and, in fact, any young man or woman entering a surgical career.

# Acknowledgments

We are indebted to:

Larry Carter
Berta Steiner
Kimberly Kist
John Gardner
Jan Thomas

# Contents

Foreword

Bradford Cannon, M.D.        vii

Mark M. Ravitch, M.D.        ix


Preface        xi

Acknowledgments        xii

Introduction        xix

Background        xix

The Role of Surgical Technique        xxi

The Scope of This Book        xxii


1.  How to Cut Skin        1

The Anatomy of Skin        3

Holding or Fixing Skin        3

The Proper Height of the Operating Table        4

Use of the Scalpel        5

Holding the Scalpel        5
  The Power Grip        5
  The Precision Grip        5
The Role of the Assistant Surgeon        6
Special Knife Blades for Cutting Skin        8

Cutting Skin Tangentially        9

Partial (Split-Thickness) Skin Sections        9
  Small Tangential Cuts in Skin        11
  Large Tangential Cuts of Skin (Split-Thickness Skin Grafts)        11
Full-Thickness Skin Grafts        16
  Use of Patterns        16
  Cutting the Graft        18
  Protection of the Graft        18

When to Cut Skin With Scissors?        20

## 2.   Skills With Scissors    23

**Varieties of Scissors    25**

**Holding the Scissors    27**

Fixation and Control—Grips    27
Position of Scissors Between Uses    28
Tactile Control With Scissors    29

**Scissors Mechanics    31**

How the Hand Produces Shear Force    31
Left-Handed Scissors    32

**When and How to Use Scissors in Surgery    32**

Functions of Scissors    32
Using the Scissors in Hilton's Maneuver    32

**Cutting Sutures With Scissors    35**

Proper Length of Suture Ends?    35
Skin Sutures    35
Buried Sutures    35
Technique of Using Scissors to Cut Sutures    36
Cutting Moving Sutures    37
Cutting Steel    38

**Use of Scissors in Combination With Other Instruments    38**

Bimanual Techniques    38
Ambidexterity    38

## 3.   How to Hold Skin    39

**Instruments Used to Hold Tissue    41**

Fingers    41
Skin Hooks    45
Forceps    46
Retractors    50
   *Types of Retractors    50*
   *Self-Retaining Retractors    50*
   *Handheld Retractors    50*
   *Suture Retraction    54*

**The Surgical Assistant's Role    57**

**The Moving Wound Principle    57**

## 4.   Dissection and Skin Undermining    59

**Which Instrument to Use?    61**

Fingertip Dissection    61
Sponge or Gauze Dissection    63

Scissors Dissection    65
Knife Dissection    65
Press Cutting    65
Laser Dissection    67
Electrocautery Dissection    67
The Hemostatic (Shaw) Scalpel    68

**Role of the Surgical Assistant    68**


**5.  Hemostasis and Removal of Blood From the Surgical Field    69**

**Historical Methods of Arresting Bleeding    71**

**Methods of Arresting Bleeding    71**

Hemostasis by Pressure    71
   *Direct Occlusion by Fingertip    71*
   *Pressure Against Underlying Bone    71*
   *Bidigital Compression (Pinch Method)    73*
   *Pressure With Knife or Instrument Tip    74*
   *Sponge and Sponge Stick Pressure    75*
   *Pressure by Packing    75*
Hemostasis by Twist Occlusion    76
Hemostasis by Ligatures and Metal Clips    76
   *Types of Ligatures    76*
   *An All-Purpose Two-Handed Tie    76*
   *Tie-on-a-Clamp    84*
   *Instrument Tie-in-a-Hole    86*
   *Metallic Clips    90*
Hemostasis by Suture Ligatures    91
   *Placing of Sutures Through Vessels    91*
   *Suture of Buried Bleeders    92*
   *Temporary Suture Tourniquet of Vessels in Continuity    92*
   *Direct Suture of Vessel Walls    94*
   *Patch Repair of Vessel Walls    94*
Hemostasis by Electrocautery    95
   *History    95*
   *Cautery Techniques    95*
Hemostasis in Bleeding Done by Vessel Plugging    97
Hemostasis With Drugs    97
   *Vasoconstrictor Drugs    97*
   *Topical Clotting Agents    98*
   *Hemostasis by Controlled Systemic Hypotension    98*
Deliberate Embolism–Intravascular Occlusion of Regional Vessels    98
   *Intra-arterial Embolism    98*
   *Intravascular Balloon Tamponade    100*

**Removing Blood and Clots From Surgical Wounds    100**

Sponging    101
Suction    102
Irrigation    104
   *Physiologic Saline    104*
   *Topical Antibiotic Solutions    106*

# 6.  Suturing Wounds    107

## Needles and Sutures    109

Handheld Needles    109
Pie-Crust Suturing of Skin Grafts    109
Selection of Needles and Needle Holders    109

## Use of the Needle Holder    112

## Suturing Skin    116

Inserting the Needle    116
Obtaining Ideal Skin Approximation    116
Role of the Assistant    118
Tying Knots With the Needle Holder    118

## Subcuticular Sutures    122

When to Use—or Not Use    122
Placing the Knots Deep    122
Errors in Placing Subcuticular Sutures    124
Placing Subcuticular Sutures With Minimal Trauma    124
Long-Term Fate of Subcuticular Nylon    125

## The Running Intradermal Pull-Out Suture    126

Advantages    126
Technique of Placing    126

## Running Cuticular Suture    128

Advantages and Disadvantages    128
Technique    128
Use of a Running Suture to Affix a Skin Graft to the Margins of a Wound    133

## Mattress Sutures    134

Indications, Advantages, and Disadvantages    134
Vertical Mattress Sutures    134
Horizontal Mattress Sutures    134

## Retention or "Stay" Sutures    135

When Indicated?    135
Dangers of Retention Sutures    135
Technical Precautions    135

## Special Suturing Techniques    137

Suturing in Narrow Deep Spaces    137
Suturing With Advancement and Sewing Around Curves    138
Suturing by Bisection    140
Closure of a Skin Defect or Donor Site With Local Tissues    140

## Proper Tension on Sutures    142

History    142
Judging Tension    143

Setting Proper Knot Tension    144
  *Silk    144*
  *Synthetic Suture Materials    148*
  *Absorbable Sutures    148*
  *Metallic Sutures    149*

## Role of the Surgical Assistant in Suturing    149

Who Will Tie the Knots? Who Will Cut the Sutures?    150
Needle Fixation and Presentation    152
Anticipating Needs for Drains and Dressings    153
Discussing Postoperative Management and Dangers    154
Educational Activities During the Operation    154

# 7.  Dressings, Drains, and Suture Removal    155

## Dressings—Art or Skill?    157

## Purposes of Dressings and Drains    157

Wound Protection    157
Promotion of Wound Drainage    158
Dressings Intended to Kill Wound Bacteria    159
Dressings That Splint the Wound    159
  *Splinting of Skin Grafts    160*
  *Plaster of Paris Casts and Other Rigid External Dressings    162*
  *Splinting of One Structure to Protect Another    163*
  *Splinting of Painful Joints or Muscles    163*
  *Dressings That Elevate a Body Part    163*
Dressings That Reduce Tension on Healing Wounds    163
  *Adhesive Skin Tapes    164*
  *The Logan Bow    165*
Pressure Dressings    167
  *Nonelastic Dressings    167*
  *Elastic Dressings    167*
Dressings for Psychological or Aesthetic Needs    167

## Drains    168

Differing Views    168
Reasons for Draining a Wound    168
Management of Postoperative Hematoma    168
When to Drain?    168
Open Versus Closed Drainage    170
  *Open Drainage    170*
  *Closed Suction Drainage    170*

## Suture Removal    171

Techniques of Suture Removal    171
  *Removing Interrupted Sutures    172*
  *Special Instruments    174*
  *Removing Running Sutures    174*
Timing of Suture Removal    174
Skin Fixation to Replace Sutures    175
  *Adhesive Skin Tapes    175*
  *Collodion Gauze Patches    176*

## 8. Special Surgical Techniques; Operating Room Hand Signals; The Left-Handed Surgeon    177

**Alloplastic Implants in Surgery    179**

**Bone Carpentry    180**

**Removal of "Dog Ears" in Closing Skin    182**

**Razabrasion and Dermabrasion    186**

**Pinch Testing for Motor Nerve Identification    186**

**Injection Techniques With Local Anesthesia    188**

**The Left-Handed Surgeon    191**

**Hand Signals in the Operating Room    191**

**Index    211**

# Introduction

Hippocrates (460–380 B.C.) discovered many of the secrets of good surgical technique. He wrote about the level of the patient's position, the proper location for the surgeon, the need for keeping the surgeon's hands and nails clean and scrubbed and the importance of boiling water before using it to wash wounds.

Much of the surgical knowledge of Hippocrates was soon lost in the dark ages of European medicine. Most of his principles had to be rediscovered centuries later. We would hope that this painful process of relearning will not have to be repeated again.

—Remarks by the author in a lecture to medical students on basic surgery, October 1987.

## Background

In the first half of the 20th century throughout the United States, the major responsibility for teaching basic or "core" surgical skills was assumed by the postgraduate training programs in general surgery. Often this teaching was excellent. Many general surgery residency programs included extensive junior resident rotations that would allow the neophyte surgeon to spend varying periods of time observing and assisting surgeons in the operating rooms of most of the surgical specialties. During each rotation, the basic concepts and skills of that particular surgical discipline were demonstrated. The quality of this training was further strengthened by the fact that most senior general surgeons in the United States during the 1930s, 1940s, and 1950s were broadly experienced both in general surgery and in surgery that involved many specialty disciplines. As a result, this author was exposed to strong emphasis on the basic handling of tissue in his surgical training at The Barnes Hospital in St. Louis, at The Valley Forge General Hospital in Pennsylvania, and at The Johns Hopkins Hospital in Baltimore.

I have had the pleasure of heading two major university residency teaching programs in plastic surgery: from 1951 to 1970 at The Johns Hopkins Hospital and between 1970 and 1987 at The University of Virginia Medical Center in Charlottesville. During these periods, many fine young surgeons rotated onto the plastic surgery service from general surgery and from most of the other surgical specialties. It has been satisfying to witness the delight and enthusiasm of many of these young residents as they first became aware of a better or simpler way to use a particular surgical instrument. Any fresh insight into the practical reasons for manipulating tissue in a particular fashion that improves the surgical result, gives any surgeon a sense of satisfaction and generates enthusiasm for his trade. Many of these former surgical residents now head their own teaching programs in major hospitals and clinics around the world. A number have stated, in subsequent years, how much they still use and value those elementary principles of surgical technique which they learned while serving a junior rotation as a resident on plastic surgery.

This book is primarily addressed to any surgeon who has an intellectual curiosity about the detailed manual activities of his trade. The Greek word for surgeon is "chirugeon"—literally, "the hand." There is no profession or trade in which the proper use of the hand is more central or important than in surgery.

Optimal surgical techniques depend on—and are limited by—the anatomical and physiological peculiarities of the human hand and eye, the functioning of our central and peripheral nervous systems, and the fortunate circumstance that the physiology of wound healing is relatively consistent from one patient to the next. Many centuries hence, it is possible that evolution will have changed significantly the shape of the human hand or the number of its digits or joints. At that time new books on basic surgical techniques will be needed. Until then, the principles of handling tools and tissues that are described in this book should be valid. This book will be of no value to Martian surgeons if they turn out to have only claws or two-fingered hands.

Why a book on something so basic as the art of surgical technique at this time? During the last few decades, many hospitals have established new teaching residency programs in plastic surgery. Simultaneously, the percentage of residents entering all surgical specialties who have an opportunity to rotate onto one of these plastic surgery services has decreased steadily with each passing year. This decrease has resulted, in part, from longer training program requirements in the surgical specialties and, in part, from an increase in the specialized nature of training that is given to general surgeons. Many general surgeons (and the majority of surgeons training in other surgical specialties) *now receive almost no fundamental training in those principles of surgery that are not only critically important to plastic surgeons, but also to all other members of the surgical profession.*

Why are the principles of plastic surgery of genuine importance to all surgeons? Plastic surgery has been defined by Ravitch* as a specialty "concerned with precise and intricate manipulations of the skin and its contents." Skin is a complex organ that differs greatly from one part of the body to another. Because of its surface location, it allows direct and continuous observation of the results of any surgical manipulation performed upon it. It must always be opened and closed when surgery on deeper tissues of the body is required. It is thus a "master tissue" in teaching us the basic laws of surgical technique. If we treat it badly, the error will quickly make itself evident. The ideal methods and precautions of handling skin have proved to be of equal value when handling deeper tissues and organs. Living cells in internal organs respond to trauma in much the same way as do the cells within our skin.

The growing body of biochemical and physiological knowledge has inevitably reduced the amount of time available for teaching the manual aspects of surgery. Yet many of the tissue-handling techniques used by plastic surgeons are of considerable value to surgeons of any specialty. Orthopedic surgeons, neurosurgeons, urologists, otolaryngologists, ophthalmologists, gynecologists, cardiovascular surgeons, and pediatric surgeons, as well as general and plastic surgeons, can profit from giving thought and attention to the precise ways they move and use their hands. These movements occupy their attention in the operating rooms for many hours each day and for many years of their lives.

The emergence of the specialty of family practice, with its emphasis on providing continuity of care, including care of many minor surgical problems, suggests that even some nonsurgical physicians may find a book on basic surgery to be of value.

---

*Mark Ravitch, M.D., personal communication.

# The Role of Surgical Technique

Teaching young surgeons how to handle tissues in a gentle and efficient fashion is one of the most important goals in surgical education. Sound knowledge regarding the diagnosis and pathogenesis of disease must be coupled with seasoned judgment and precise execution if a surgical operation is to give the patient an optimum result. Once the decision to operate has been properly made, the correct handling of surgical instruments and tissues will do much to minimize damage and accelerate healing. Roughness in the handling of tissue or the use of crushing instruments may lead to disastrous surgical complications and even death.

All surgery may be viewed as various combinations of "cutting, sewing, and tying." The surgeon uses metallic instruments (or electrical or light energy) to cut through the many layers of the human body. Instruments improve his grasp on tissues, help him find his way beneath the depths of the wound, and help him obtain an unobstructed view of his working field. Suction tips and sponges remove blood and fluids. An electric cautery, laser, or bone wax seals the open ends of bleeding vessels. Needles, holders, and sutures may then reapproximate the tissues.

Nonetheless, most of these surgical instruments serve only as specialized extensions of the surgeon's hands and fingers. The best and most useful instruments are often the simplest in design. The only instrument that possesses the marvelous quality of tactile sensation is the surgeon's hand itself. *His finest tools are his fingertips!*

This book stresses the most basic aspects of surgical technique—namely, the precise ways in which the surgeon communicates with the tissues. It is the goal of any surgeon to open the skin, to carry out the indicated physical rearrangement of internal parts, and then to retreat, *having disturbed the normal physiology as little as possible*. He wants to leave his patient with a wound that has the maximum chance for prompt and kindly healing.

Fortunately, much basic surgical technique can be taught with the aid of simple, clear illustrations. In bringing this surgical technique atlas into being, I was fortunate to have had the help of Ms. Florence Kabir, a talented and conscientious medical artist and photographer, and of Williams & Wilkins, a medical publisher known for its stress on quality reproduction of illustrations. We hope this book will be a joy and an aid to many young doctors during their surgical careers. Some may find it of special help during their first years of postgraduate residency training.

Even surgeons with much experience may enjoy the opportunity this book may offer to reflect on their own manual skills and perhaps suggest to them points of instruction that they may share with their younger associates. During the writing of this book, I have certainly enjoyed coming to understand better my own movements and methods within the operating room.

While it is true that beautiful surgical technique will not produce a fine result if the wrong operation is chosen, it is equally true that excellent handling of tissue improves the results of any operation.

# 1
## How to Cut Skin

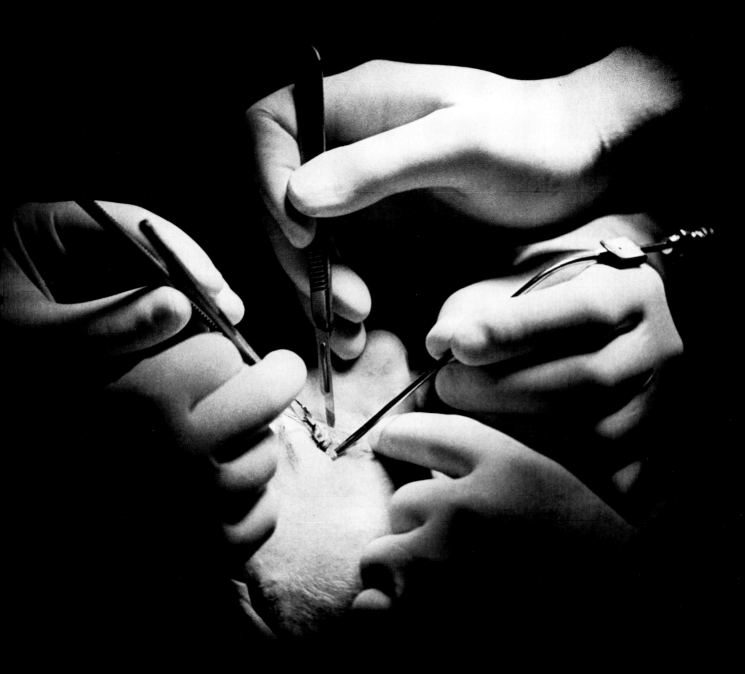

# 1
## How to Cut Skin

## The Anatomy of Skin

The skin of the human eyelid is only 0.6 mm thick. Yet it is twenty times that thick over the back of the same person! The dermis of the skin is composed of a tough waterproof weave of collagen and elastic fibers. A sharp knife and significant force are required to part it cleanly. A dull knife is dangerous and causes unnecessary damage when used to cut the dermis. Since most skin is only loosely attached to the underlying tissues, it must first be held and stabilized in order to cut it accurately.

## Holding or Fixing Skin

Skin is mobile over the underlying bones and muscles, thanks to the interposition, in most parts of the body, of one or more layers of subcutaneous fat and fascia containing attenuated vertical attachments to the skin. Thus, the accurate cutting of skin requires deliberate external fixation of this tough but mobile integument so that the scalpel blade will incise it cleanly and vertically in the intended fashion.

Skin fixation may be obtained by the surgeon or his assistant if he will place his hands on either side of the intended incision. The skin is first pressed firmly downward, and the hands or fingers are then spread apart from one another to provide a tight stretching of the area to be incised. Once the surgeon places the blade of the scalpel against the skin, the assistant's hands should remain absolutely immobile until the knife is again lifted away from the tissues. If the stabilizing hands of the assistant should shift, even slightly, while the knife is in motion, an inaccurate or beveled incision will result. If the skin is moist or oily, its fixation by the assistant or the surgeon is further aided by placing a dry gauze sponge on the skin before spreading it.

When the first assistant is not familiar with the surgeon's routines, or if he fails to exercise helpful initiatives, the surgeon will often fix the skin surface himself with his nondominant hand (Fig. 1.1).

Using the pulp of his left thumb, the surgeon presses the skin on the near side of the incision back toward himself, and thus toward the near side of the operating table. The pulps of his index and long fingers simultaneously press the far side of the intended line of incision to spread the skin away from the thumb and toward the far side of the table. With the skin so fixed, the knife is placed equidistant between the thumb and fingertips, and the incision is made with a firm, smooth, and definite stroke. Note that in Figure 1.1 the scalpel is held in the right hand in the manner most commonly used by the general surgeon. The handle is gripped firmly between the pulp of the right thumb and the flexed proximal interphalangeal joint of the index finger. The midportion of the scalpel handle lies beneath the head of the third metacarpal and gains further support from contact with the palm in the region of the heads of the fourth and fifth metacarpals. The long, ring, and little fingers are flexed around the handle so as to control both the angle and rotation of the blade. Accurate positioning of the edge of the knife blade is accomplished by flexion, extension, and rotation of the wrist, and *not* by shifting of the fingers and thumb. This method of gripping the scalpel allows the surgeon to exert considerable downward force on the skin. Both the epidermis and dermis should be incised completely with the initial stroke.

When making very long incisions, the surgeon pauses in his cutting stroke as soon as he feels any undesirable increase in the lateral mobility of the tissues beneath his moving knife blade. He should pause with his knife stroke while he repositions his nondominant hand forward to a point just beyond the already completed part of the skin incision. The skin is spread and fixed once again by the fingers and thumb, and the knife is again pressed downward and then forward to extend the cut for the desired additional distance. This process is repeated until the entire incision has been made.

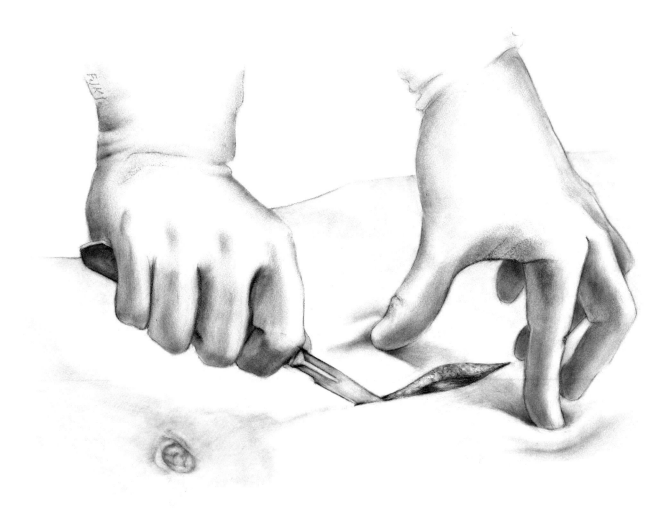

**Figure 1.1**

## Proper Height of the Operating Table

Occasionally, surgeons will be seen operating with the table and operating field at much too high a level. This may result from an unconscious desire to bring the operating field closer to the eyes in the hope of improving vision. In the absence of uncorrected myopia, this error should be avoided. Once the operating field reaches the level of the surgeon's elbows, any further elevation requires a significant compensatory flexing of the wrists. Figure 1.2A shows the ideal level of the operating table when about to make an incision on the abdomen or chest. Note that the surgeon's wrist is in slight dorsiextension—the ''position of ideal function.''

When the table is above elbow level, wrist flexion automatically tightens the long extensor and relaxes the long flexor tendons in the forearms and hands. Figure 1.2B shows the table too high, causing the surgeon to increase flexion of both his elbows and his wrists. In that position, the long flexor and long extensor tendons to his fingers are no longer in tonic balance. This imbalance reduces small muscle control within the hands and increases fatigue. Eye stereopsis is also more accurate if the operating table is low enough to keep the operative field at least 18 inches from the eyes.

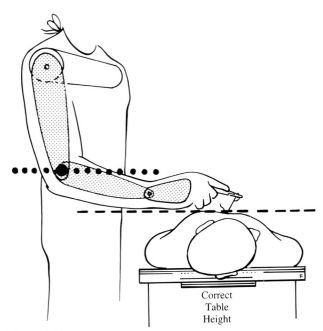

Correct
Table
Height

**Figure 1.2A**

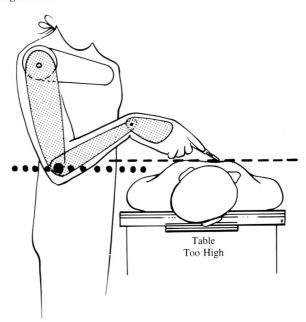

Table
Too High

**Figure 1.2B**

When the surgeon is forced to operate on a depressed body surface, or within the mouth or a body cavity, the operating field should be well *below* the level of the surgeon's elbows. This allows him to keep his wrists relatively straight or in slight dorsal extension and mild ulnar deviation. This position is the "functional position" of the wrist, and it greatly improves dexterity and strength in the fingers. The skilled surgeon will avoid a table height that requires him to work with his wrists in a position of flexion.

## Use of the Scalpel

### Holding the Scalpel

There are two basic methods of holding the scalpel: the power grip and the precision grip.

**The power grip**

The power grip has been described above (Fig. 1.1) and is the one most commonly used by the general surgeon, the cardiovascular surgeon, or the gynecologist. Note that the shaft of the scalpel is braced against the palm of the hand, and that portion of the handle which is just behind the blade is grasped in a key pinch position between the pulp of the thumb and the radial side of the flexed proximal interphalangeal joint of the index finger. This key pinch prevents the blade from turning while the palm and remaining fingers are used to apply the needed downward force to the skin.

The power grip of the scalpel is designed to allow the surgeon to incise completely through large distances in the dermis and epidermis quickly and accurately with a single stroke. With increasing experience, the layer of subcutaneous fat may also be divided with the initial cut. But take care! One well-known general surgeon presses so firmly on the knife that he frequently divides the rectus abdominis fascia with his first stroke, and on occasion he has been known to incise the lobe of the liver with that initial passage of his blade! Needless to say, this is not considered good form.

The assistant should attempt to stretch and fix the skin with the aid of sponges before the surgeon positions the blade of his knife in preparation for the incision. *The assistant should not relax this skin tension until the surgeon pauses in his stroke or lifts the scalpel.* If the assistant should tighten or loosen the skin while the knife is cutting, a beveled or misdirected incision may result. Long incisions may require two or three resettings of the assistant's hands to improve skin fixation and the accuracy of cut. The surgeon should avoid the use of multiple shallow strokes of the scalpel to penetrate the dermis. This will only add more trauma, take more time, and delay healing.

**The precision grip**

When the surgeon wishes to use a scalpel to cut skin in an angular or curving fashion with maximum accuracy, the power grip is not suitable. This is especially true if the skin to be incised is very thin, if the cut must be precisely curved, or if there are sharp angles that require the surgeon to change the direction of the knife stroke. In such circumstances the precision grip used so commonly by plastic surgeons gives greater control.

In Figure 1.3 the surgeon is using a precision grip. The scalpel is held much in the manner in which a writer holds a pen, or a painter a fine brush. The handle of the scalpel is supported by allowing it to rest loosely on the dorsum of the web between the thumb and index finger. The grooved portion of the scalpel handle is held by three-point fixation between the pulps of the thumb and index fingers, with the third point being the radial aspect of the distal interphalangeal joint of the long finger. This third point of support also lies just beneath that part of the scalpel handle which is held between the pulps of the thumb and index finger.

Additional stabilization is provided by a point of contact with the patient by the tip of the long finger. At times, this contact point is a resting site for the ulnar side of the ring or little finger. Patient-hand contact steadies the position of the knife edge in the surgeon's hand and allows a light grip of the handle by the thumb and index finger. This makes it easier to turn the moving blade from side to side, as the surgeon selects the exact angle and positioning of the knife edge. The long finger, and sometimes the ring and little fingers, are thus deliberately placed in contact with the patient in order to stabilize the operator's knife hand. Such contact keeps the knife hand from being airborne and allows the surgeon to relax the large muscles in the forearm and upper arm. A score of beautifully coordinated small intrinsic muscles within the hand are thereby freed to give maximum dexterity to the fingers.

Note also in Figure 1.3 how the surgeon has placed some gauze beneath the fingertips of his left hand to get better traction on a moist skin surface. Meanwhile, the assistant's left hand is maintaining fixation of the skin on the opposite side of the incision. This hand remains motionless as the surgeon selects the desired curve of his cut.

Many neophyte surgeons have difficulty in holding their hands and instruments steady when they first begin to work in the operating room. Sometimes they believe themselves to be "too nervous" for a career in surgery. In almost every case, tremor of the hands may be cured by showing the resident how to brace and relax the large muscles of the forearms. Bracing the hands or arms by resting them lightly against some

part of the field or the patient avoids the increase in muscle tone that is required to support the hand in a midair position. Arm relaxation is one of the most effective ways of eliminating hand tremor. *The relaxed arm gives a steady hand!* Those engaged in microsurgery have learned this lesson and find the use of metal arm rests invaluable when operating under magnifications of 6 to 40 powers.

For both the power grip and the precision grip of the scalpel, it is mandatory that the skin surface be fixed firmly in position before cutting. The operator will use his nondominant hand to fix the skin and provide counterforce to the pull of the knife (Fig. 1.3).

## The Role of the Assistant Surgeon

An alert and sensitive first assistant surgeon will anticipate where the incision into the skin is to be made. He will be ready to use his hands to fix the tissues before the surgeon actually places the knife. If the skin surface is moist, a dry gauze sponge will improve traction on the skin (Fig. 1.3). The assistant should not wait for the surgeon to request him to fix the skin. Good surgical teamwork requires that the assistant be constantly alert. He must anticipate the sequence of surgical steps and try to stay ahead of the surgeon in planning the next phase of the operation. He should take pride in seeing how often he can be in position and ready to facilitate the operation without being given specific instructions. When surgeons work together over a period of time, teamwork becomes much more efficient and few words need be spoken.

Whenever the surgeon is concentrating on the immediate task at hand, it is of great value if the first assistant addresses some of his attention to the overall situation. He should ask himself certain questions: Does the field have adequate light? Are the wound margins properly retracted? Should any bleeding be controlled at that moment? Is the field free of loose instruments and bits of suture material? Is the second assistant positioned properly and using his hands effectively? Does the scrub nurse have ready the instruments and sutures that will be needed next? Does the patient's EKG monitor show a normal pattern? Is the patient's blood bright red or dark? Is there any exposed tissue that could be temporarily protected by covering it with moist saline sponges? These and numerous other questions should continuously occupy the thoughts of any good first assistant. The key words are to *anticipate* and *facilitate*. There is no place at

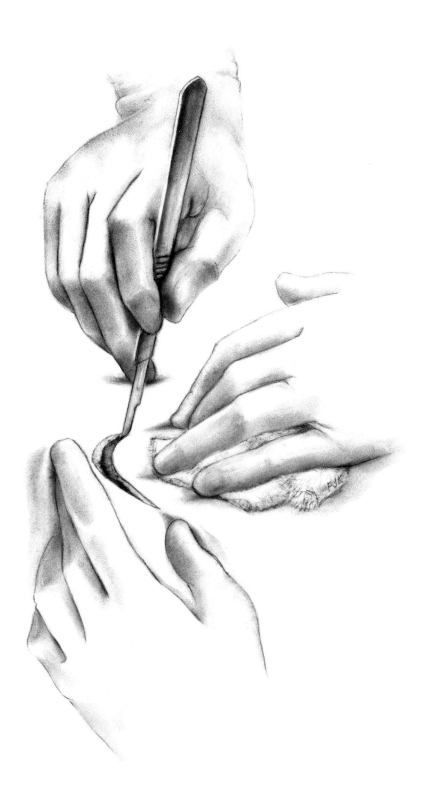

**Figure 1.3**

the operating table for an assistant who periodically develops the glazed look of someone in a "catatonic trance." An assistant should feel embarrassed if the surgeon frequently needs to take the initiative in many of these support maneuvers.

The late Sterling Bunnell would sometimes greet his surgical assistants in the morning with the joking salutation, "Good morning, opponents numbers one and two." The good surgical assistant strives to conduct himself so that such a salutation will only be in jest. A poor or inattentive assistant will make even the best surgeon look inept in the operating room.

Most surgeons encourage their assistants to ask appropriate questions during an operation. Such questions show active thought and interest. However, the timing of the question is important, and questions about a future step in the operation which might be answered by the reply, "Stick around and see,"

should be avoided. The assistant would do well to read about the operation the night before if he is unfamiliar with the condition or planned operation. He should always review the regional anatomy before each procedure. The alert and informed assistant will usually be given more operative responsibilities at an early stage of his training than one who is only "doing his job."

### Special Knife Blades for Cutting Skin

At times, the use of a scalpel blade of special shape will aid the surgeon. I have found that only a few of the many available blade shapes are of value with any reasonable frequency.

The #11 scalpel blade tapers to a very fine point. This slender point is of special value in excising very small skin lesions when full-thickness removal of the skin is necessary (Fig. 1.4). The sharp point will allow

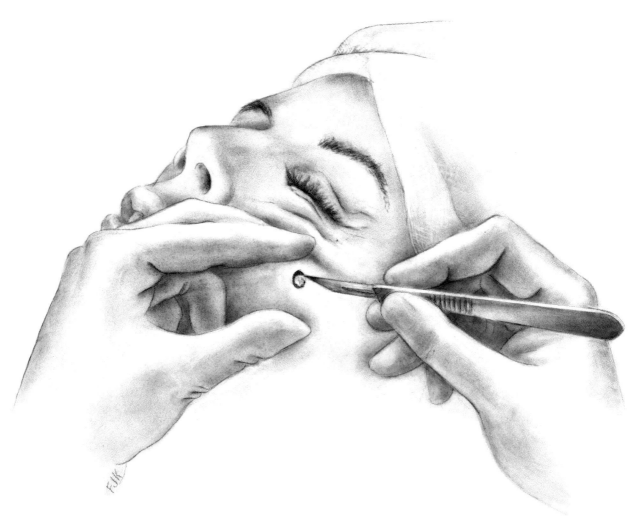

**Figure 1.4**

the surgeon to change direction easily to produce tight curves and angles. Care must be taken not to insert this blade too far, as the fine tip will often be found to have reached a deeper level than the surgeon expected. When using a #11 blade, care is taken to maintain gentle but constant and steadily advancing pressure against the blade edge throughout the to-and-fro sawing motions of the knife. If any letup in this pressure occurs, an irregularity or notching of the incised skin margin will result. As with all scalpel cuts, the skin should be firmly fixed with the opposite hand before inserting the point of the blade. In Figure 1.4 the surgeon is using a #11 blade to remove a small nevus of the cheek. Before inserting the knife blade, the skin is fixed by pinching a fold of it upward tightly between the thumb and index fingers of the operator's left hand. This provides both fixation and hemostasis during the cutting.

Right-angled scalpel blades (Fig. 1.5A) are only required for very special purposes in surgery. Such blades may be of help when a cut must be made into tissue that is at the bottom of a hole or along the walls of a deep cavity of small diameter. At such times, the cut must be made at right angles to the long axis of the scalpel handle. Plastic surgeons, ophthalmologists, otolaryngologists, and neurosurgeons periodically find good use for right-angled blades. Figure 1.5B shows the details of the straight, more commonly used #11 blade.

A #12 blade combines the features of a sharp pointed tip with a crescent-shaped cutting edge of the blade (Fig. 1.5C). The sharp edge lies along the concave margin of the crescent. This blade shape may be of value when a cut must be made back toward the surgeon within a deep hole or cavity. The knife tip may be inserted into tissue and the cut made by pulling the blade back toward the surface. At times this blade may be used to divide dangling or mobile tissue by inserting the tip and pushing it away from the point of entrance. The curve of the blade allows the surgeon first to impale the tissue with the tip, while the continued pressure of the cutting edge of the blade maintains tissue fixation and stretch until the incision is completed. The #12 blade is rarely used to cut skin.

## Cutting Skin Tangentially

Surgeons often cut skin in a plane parallel to its surface. This may be necessary to remove unsightly or dangerous cutaneous lesions that do not extend into the underlying subcutaneous tissue. At other times, sheets or segments of normal skin may be removed from one part of the body to provide a graft for resurfacing of a second area.

These tangential cuts of skin may be at either partial-thickness or full-thickness depths. The methods of cutting are quite different for these different thicknesses.

### Partial (Split-Thickness) Skin Sections

At times, the surgeon will need to cut skin so that only the epidermis and part of the dermis are removed. In such cases, some of the deep dermis is retained and healing occurs by epithelialization. Such healing requires no suturing and avoids the type of scar formation that always follows cuts or incisions that penetrate the full thickness of the dermis.

Because the dermis of human skin is extremely tough, any knife edge that cuts tangentially at the level of the deep dermis will tend to be diverted, either superficially or more deeply, as it seeks an easier (less dense) plane. For this reason, a knife edge of superior sharpness is required for splitting skin tangentially.

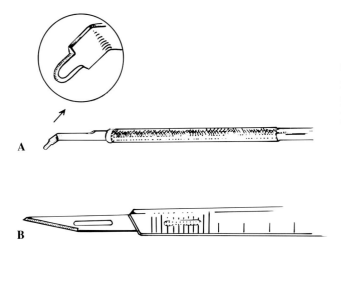

**Figure 1.5**

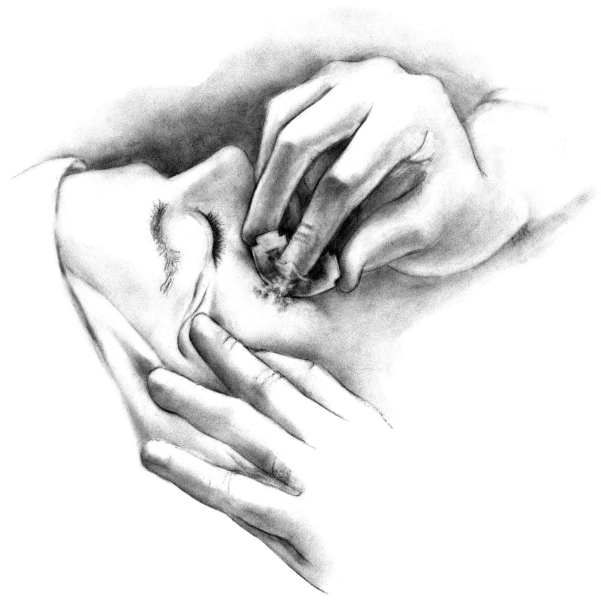

**Figure 1.6**

**Small tangential cuts in skin**

Small skin lesions or birthmarks may be removed with an ordinary double-edged razor blade. Tangential excision is particularly useful in parts of the body where the skin is relatively thick. This technique is known as razabrasion and requires a bit of practice (on an orange). As shown in Figure 1.6, an ordinary double-edged razor blade is bent into a curve by the thumb and long fingers and braced in this position by downward pressure with the pulp of the index finger. The nevus or lesion to be removed is placed under firm stretch by fixing the surrounding skin. The razor is then used to shave off the lesion by using alternating supination and pronation circular motions of the wrist to advance the cutting edge. The direction of these motions should follow the curve of the bend in the razor. I prefer to start the excision at a very superficial depth several millimeters behind the edge of the lesion. The cut is deepened (using visual monitoring) and progressively widened (by reducing the amount of blade flex) as the razor passes beneath the center of the lesion at sufficient depth to include the desired thickness of dermis on the deep side of the lesion, along with the removed specimen. An additional thin layer of deep dermis remains below the cut. On emerging at the far side of the lesion, the edge of the razor is allowed gradually to come up to a superficial level by reducing downward pressure on the blade. This tapers the depth of the cut of all margins of the excised area and improves the final scar. No sutures are required. The area is dressed with fine mesh gauze or telfa.

Razabrasion is an extremely valuable method for tangential cutting of skin. The use of a flexible and bowed razor blade allows the surgeon to use this method, even on concave areas of the body surface, by simply increasing or decreasing the bend in the blade to match the curve of the skin surface. Straight razors do not offer this advantage. Straight or bowed knife edges may be used in this same fashion to harvest small split-thickness skin grafts for use in repair of small traumatic defects. Razabrasion is not of value in areas where the skin is very thin such as the eyelids or the lateral surfaces of the ears.

**Large tangential cuts of skin
(split-thickness skin grafts)**

Removal of large tangential sections of skin may be required in many situations. The most common indication is the harvesting of split-thickness skin grafts to cover an open wound on another part of the body. The method is also of value in resurfacing after removal of giant pigmented nevi in infants, in removing unwanted ornamental tattoos, and in the tangential débridement of necrotic burned skin following thermal injury. Two basically different methods exist for cutting large sheets of skin tangentially.

The Free-Hand Knife

Vilray Blair and Ferris Smith were among the first to advocate use of a long, flat sharp knife to slice skin tangentially. This was originally accomplished without the aid of shims or protective guards. The Ferris Smith knife is shown in Figure 1.7. Its special feature was the use of a replaceable 6-inch blade. The blade is removed by sliding it out of the groove in the firm metal arm that continues as an extension of the handle. The small round metal plate at the base of the blade serves as a convenient resting spot for the pulp of the surgeon's index finger. The method requires the surgeon to engage in some practice but is a useful skill that is readily acquired.

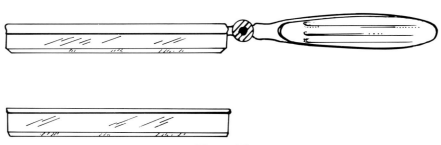

**Figure 1.7**

As shown in Figure 1.8, the skin of the thigh, buttock or other appropriate donor area is first flattened and stretched between a wooden board and a small rectangular metallic suction box. The board is pressed against one end of the chosen donor site by an assistant, but the suction box is held in the non-dominant hand of the surgeon. The surfaces of the skin and the knife blade are lubricated with a thin layer of mineral oil to reduce friction or drag against the moving knife blade. The operator then slices the skin exactly as one would slice a thin sheet of ham or salmon.

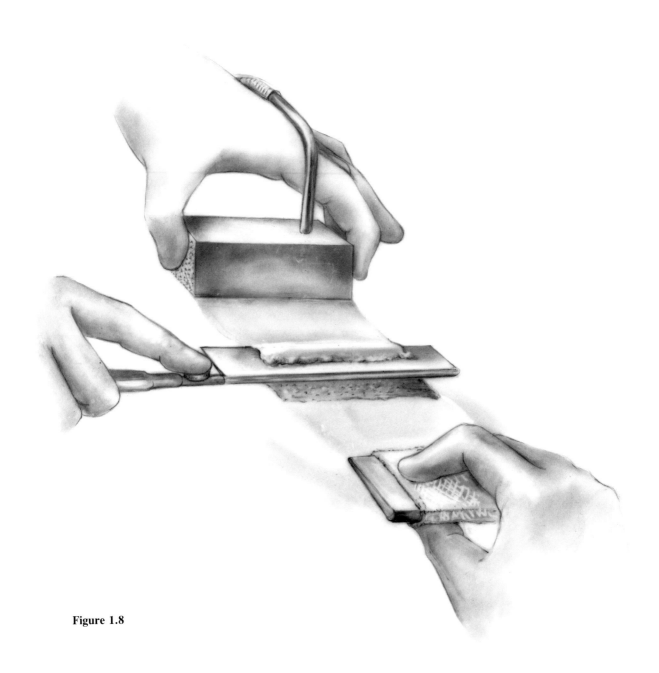

**Figure 1.8**

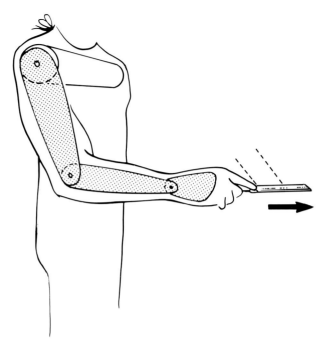

**Figure 1.9A**

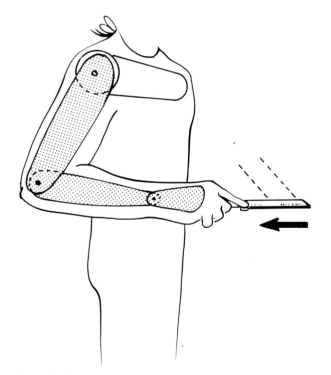

**Figure 1.9B**

The motion is a relaxed free-swinging action of shoulder and elbow with a fixed position of the hand and wrist (Fig. 1.9A–B). Note that the wrist-hand-knife unit remains fixed at both ends of the stroke. This swing should be smooth and relatively rapid. The stroke should travel the full length of the knife edge. The surgeon should be aware of exerting some down-

ward pressure with the flat of the knife blade (but with no sense of pushing forward its cutting edge) against the donor site. Increasing or decreasing this downward pressure will allow him to make the skin graft either thicker or thinner as the cutting proceeds.

There should be no conscious effort by the surgeon to push the knife edge forward. All advancing of the blade occurs by the almost unconscious shifting of the surgeon's body and arm. If a forward push is attempted with the hand, the knife edge will immediately cut too deeply—or not deeply enough. This will spoil the uniformity of the graft. The cutting of the skin thus occurs equally on the push and pull strokes. Cutting only on the push stroke will cause ridges and uneven thickness in the graft.

If the skin of the donor area becomes too mobile during the cutting of the graft, the surgeon stops, and the assistant advances the fixation board to a position closer to the cutting area. The suction box is then returned to the skin 1 to 2 inches ahead of the knife edge, and the smooth swinging of the knife begins again, always keeping even downward pressure against the donor area with the flat of the moving blade.

The suction box is held in the surgeon's non-dominant hand and is slowly but continuously moved forward as the skin graft is cut. The operator strives to keep the suction box several inches in advance of the cutting knife edge. The purpose of the suction box is to flatten and lift the skin as the knife edge follows just behind. Wider suction boxes are used when wider grafts are needed.

Special guards have been designed that may be attached to the blades of some models of free-hand graft knives (such as the Humby knife), but these are not necessary and generally best left off, once some skill has been acquired.

With a modest amount of practice, the surgeon can use the free-hand skin graft knife to harvest large single split-thickness skin grafts 100 to 200 square inches in area from donor surfaces such as the thigh and buttocks. The constant visual control of the cutting edge of the knife that the free-hand graft-cutting technique provides will allow the surgeon to continuously monitor the thickness of the skin being removed. He may easily learn to vary the graft thickness between 0.008 and 0.035 inch, depending on the needs of the intended recipient site. This visual control minimizes the danger of excessively deep cuts that might produce permanent scarring of the donor area.

Once again, during the cutting of the graft, the thickness of the skin is controlled by varying the amount of downward pressure on the flat of the blade and *not* by changing the angle of the cutting edge.

The free-hand technique of cutting skin grafts is being taught less commonly in recent years. This is unfortunate as it offers many advantages over the use of dermatome machines. Since no skin glue, cement, or electricity is required, it remains the method of choice in cutting split-thickness skin grafts in the unsophisticated operating rooms that are often found in countries that have warm and humid climates. Such climates delay the "setting up" of most skin glues and make uncertain the adhesiveness and uniformity of grafts that may be obtained with most nonmotorized dermatomes. Throughout the world, skin grafts must be taken in operating rooms that lack even electric power.

Other advantages of the free-hand knife technique include the ability to cut wider and longer grafts, better control and observation of thickness of grafts in the act of cutting, reduced operating time, and more rapid donor site healing.

Dermatomes

Since the introduction of the first aluminum half-circle drum dermatome by Earl Padgett in the 1940s, surgeons have continued to devise and further improve machines for the cutting of split-thickness skin grafts. Padgett's original aluminum drum was painted with a coating of rubber cement. The engineer, Hood, suggested this method of making the skin of the patient's donor area adhere to the drum. By rolling the drum upward the skin, adherent to the rubber cement, was elevated from the body surface. The partial thickness skin graft was cut free from the donor area by to and fro strokes of a knife edge mounted on each side of the drum on two metal arms slightly longer than the radius of the curve of the half-drum. The blade was set so that its edge would stroke parallel to the curving surface of the drum. The thickness of the skin graft was determined by a caliper gauge that set the knife edge an exact distance away from the drum surface.

The Reece dermatome was invented a few years later and is shown in Figure 1.10. It is left mounted on its stand (Fig. 1.10A) until the canvas tape, thickness shim, and blade have been inserted.

The canvas-backed tape that is fitted to the drum before each use is coated with a green adhesive cover. This green tape sticks firmly to a second special (red) cement, which is painted on the skin of the patient's donor area and allowed to dry for 5 minutes before cutting. In Figure 1.10B the canvas tape has already been mounted in the slots in two steel cylinders at each end of the curved steel drum (*a*). The hand crank (*c*) is in position to tighten and flatten it against the

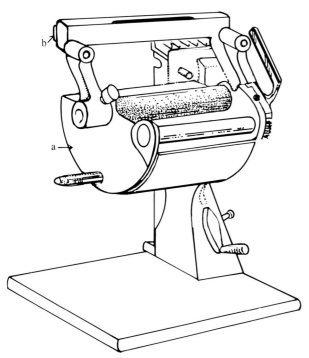

**Figure 1.10A**

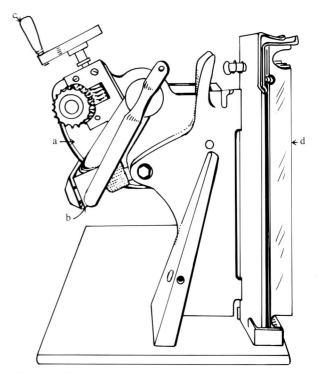

**Figure 1.10B**

curved surface of the metal drum. Caution should be taken not to tighten this crank excessively, as the rigid canvas layer within the tape may break (this is detectable only by an unexplained easing of resistance to turning of the hand crank during tightening). Should this happen and go unrecognized, it will spoil the graft removal. A new tape should be substituted.

In using the Reece dermatome, the graft thickness is determined by the use of one of a series of metal spacers or shims that are shown mounted on the side of the dermatome stand (d in Fig. 1.10B). The shim of proper thickness is chosen and placed alongside the dermatome blade in the blade clamp. This shim separates the knife edge an exact distance from the drum corresponding to the desired thickness of the graft to be cut.

The operator then removes the half-circle drum from the stand and presses its leading edge against skin surface of the donor area that has been coated with glue. The Reece dermatome was an improvement over the original Padgett machine as it was made of stainless steel, and it retains a more precise alignment of drum and blade even after repeated use.

Whenever a dermatome is used to remove skin from concave or undulating areas of the body surface, such as the spaces between the ribs or the supraclavicular fossa of the neck, several hundred milliliters of physiologic saline should first be injected into the subcutaneous fat of that region to elevate any depressed areas and flatten the skin surface prior to taking the graft.

In recent years, electric and air-driven dermatomes have been popular in the skin grafting of burns (Fig. 1.11). These do not require skin glue, but work much on the principle of oscillating knives that are used to slice cheese. A light coating of mineral oil is again placed on the skin of the donor area and on the undersurface of the dermatome before starting. This reduces friction as the dermatome glides over the skin. The blade and flat leading edge of the dermatome are pressed against the skin and moved slowly forward as the blade vibrates from side to side. As shown in Figure 1.11, the front end of the dermatome is pointed downward at a 45° angle with the donor surface as cutting proceeds. If the already-cut portion of the emerging skin graft gathers in folds over the front end of the dermatome so as to block vision, an assistant should lift it up lightly with two pairs of forceps. When a sufficient length of skin has been cut, the dermatome is angled upward to sever the last attachment of the graft.

The principal advantage of this type of dermatome is that it allows rapid harvesting of a large amount of skin. Since the donor surface must be quite flat, the blades are only about 3.5 inches wide. Consequently, this dermatome will not cut grafts as wide as those that may be obtained by the free-hand method. The length of the graft is limited only by the amount of available donor skin area that may be flattened along a straight line. Rapid harvesting of skin is of special importance in treating patients with large burns so as to shorten the duration of anesthesia time.

Dermatomes sometimes give surgeons an unwarranted sense of confidence. The thickness of the skin being removed may be unintentionally altered as the cutting proceeds if the surgeon happens to vary the pressure of the dermatome against the donor area. Dullness of the knife edge, changing the angle at which the dermatome meets the skin, or even modest lateral tilting of the machine (so as to put more pressure along one edge of the dermatome then the other) will also change graft thickness. Dermatomes are capricious, and it is best that a surgeon become familiar with a given instrument and then try to use that one machine each time he cuts a graft. In tropical and

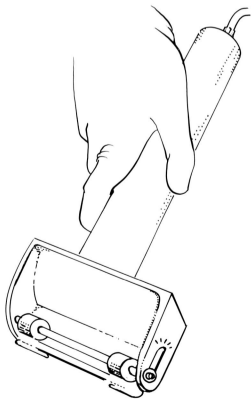

**Figure 1.11**

humid climates, the skin adhesives needed for some dermatomes are slow to dry and may also prove unreliable in lifting the skin.

## Full-Thickness Skin Grafts

Since the introduction of full-thickness skin grafting (free transplants of both the epidermis and the entire thickness of the dermis), surgeons have tried many methods of removing the full-thickness skin from donor areas. The resulting donor sites should not be expected to heal by simple epithelialization. Closure of the defect requires advancement and suture of the remaining local skin or, in the case of very large grafts, the application of a second graft of split-thickness skin taken from another donor site.

**Use of patterns**

Full-thickness skin grafts provide high-quality resurfacing, but they are of limited supply. To avoid waste, they are best cut exactly to the size and shape required. An effective aid is the preparation of a pattern from a presterilized strip of developed (transparent) x-ray film. In Figure 1.12, a piece of this film has been placed over the wound or defect to be grafted, and a dye such as Berwick Blue or Brilliant Green has been used to trace a line of dashes on the x-ray film to indicate the shape of the underlying recipient bed. The pattern for the graft is next cut out of the film with stout scissors.

The resulting stiff cutout of x-ray film is transferred to the chosen donor area and pressed firmly downward into the skin for several seconds (Fig. 1.13A). This indents the skin at the edges of the pattern. Figure 1.13B shows this residual skin indentation after removing the film. This light imprint of the exact

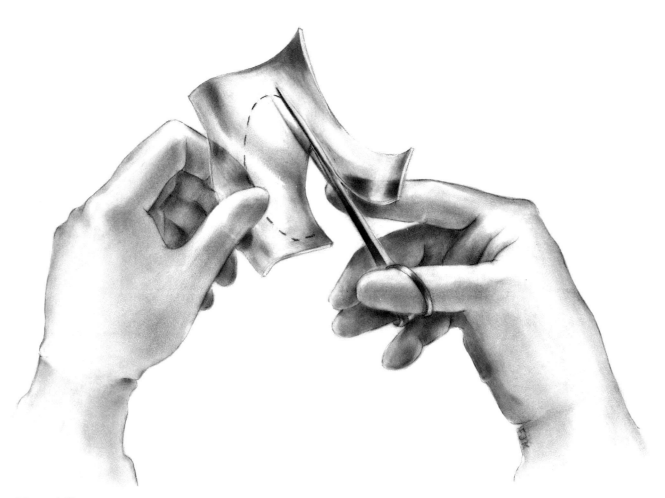

**Figure 1.12**

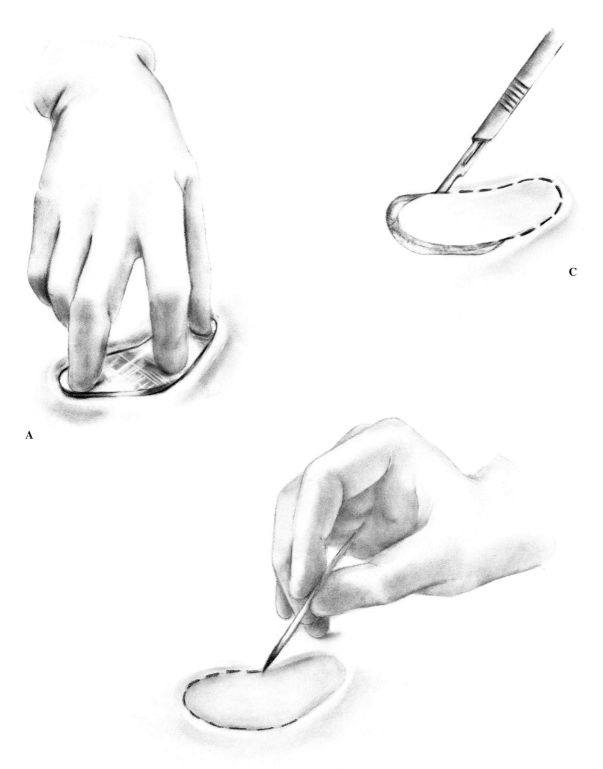

**Figure 1.13**                                    **B**

shape of the graft is then intensified by tracing over it with a toothpick dipped in the same dye used to mark the pattern on the x-ray film.

### Cutting the graft

Once marked, the entire periphery of the graft is outlined by an incision with a #15 scalpel blade, taking care to cut into—but not completely through—the dermis (Fig. 1.13C).

The success of full-thickness skin grafting depends on the complete removal of every vestige of subcutaneous fat from the deep surface of the graft. This is most easily accomplished by using the scalpel to remove the graft precisely at the level of the deep dermis. The cutting is greatly facilitated if the surgeon's assistant uses both hands to spread and fix the surrounding skin under maximum tension. The tighter the skin, the easier will be the surgical dissection.

The surgeon places a single skin hook at a convenient corner of the lightly incised graft and starts to dissect it upward. The cut should be at a depth that reveals the junction between the white layer of dermis and the deeper yellow layer of subcutaneous fat. A fresh #15 knife blade should be used. A smooth, stroking action of the knife edge will give a more uniform graft and minimize damage to the dermis. Scraping motions with the knife should be avoided, and the angle of the blade should be slightly inclined toward the dense collagen layer on the deep surface of the graft dermis. A smooth stroke will avoid ridges and variance in the graft thickness.

As the cutting proceeds, the surgeon should hold the handle of the skin hook between the thumb and index finger of his left hand (if right-handed), and the skin surface of the graft should be everted over the tip of the long finger as it is elevated with further dissection. As shown in Figure 1.14, the graft is folded outward over the tactile pulp of the long finger as the knife separates the dermis of the graft from its underlying attachments. The tip of the long finger remains in position to palpate the exact thickness of the graft as the knife continues to cut it away from the bed. Once the first corner of the graft has been well elevated, a second skin hook is positioned so that the two hooks will maintain tension and elevate both margins of the graft as they are cut free. With a little practice, the handles of both of the hooks may be easily managed in a single hand by pinching the shafts of the hooks between the thumb and index fingers and the radial side of the flexed left long finger (Fig. 1.14).

As the elevation of the graft continues, the as-sistant may feel the need to reset his fingers in order to maintain maximum tension on the surrounding skin. When this occurs, he should ask the surgeon to pause while he repositions his hands. Without this warning any release of tension may cause a misstroke of the surgeon's knife. The surgeon may also need to repeatedly shift the position of the skin hooks so as to keep their points close to those positions along the edges of the graft that are next to be elevated. This repeated resetting of the hooks also reduces prolonged and excessive graft stretching along any one axis of the graft, with consequent rupturing of its elastic and collagen fibers.

During the dissection of the graft, if care is taken to cut free the two advancing margins of the graft with the knife before dissecting up the central attachments, the operation will go more easily. If distinct punctate bleeding is encountered from the graft bed, the surgeon will know that he is cutting too deeply and dividing some of the larger subdermal blood vessels. Ideally, a thin white web of residual dermal fibers will be left covering the donor bed when the graft has been lifted.

### Protection of the graft

After removal, the deep surface of the full-thickness skin graft should be moistened with a few drops from a sponge soaked with physiological saline and inspected in a good light. Any vestiges of retained fat or mobile fascia should be trimmed away with fine dissecting scissors. This trimming or defatting process is facilitated if the operator will drape the graft upside down over the tip of his left index finger as he cuts off the tags of fat with fine scissors. The sense of thickness of the graft that is conveyed through the tip of the left index finger will minimize the danger of cutting a "buttonhole" in the graft by too deep a snip with the scissors.

The prepared graft is covered with a pad of gauze moistened with physiological saline until ready for use. The nurse should have a secure place on her back table where she may clamp the gauze containing all grafts of skin or other tissues that might be used later in the operation. A distinctive yellow or red cloth wrapper placed about the outside of the moistened sponge containing the graft will further reduce the danger of its being accidentally discarded with other used sponges. This precautionary routine becomes of considerable importance in any hospital in which scrub nurses are frequently changed during the course of a single operation.

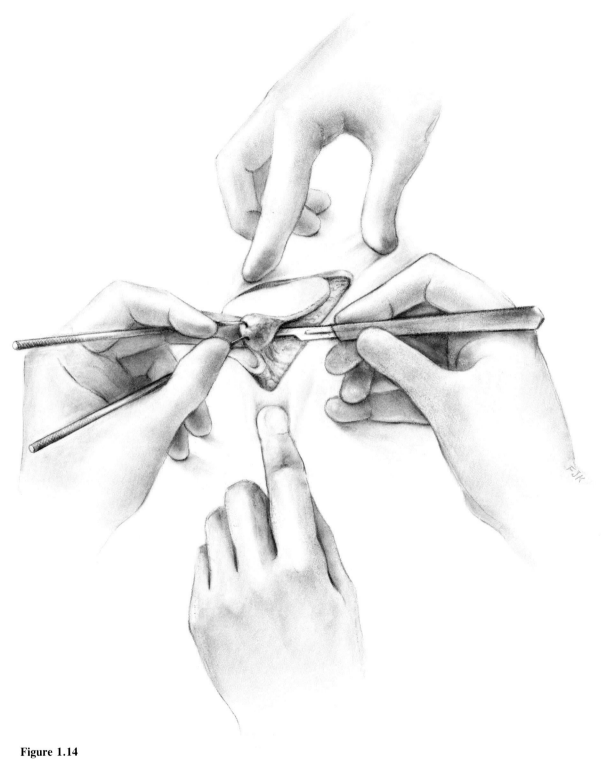

**Figure 1.14**

The preferred methods of suturing and closing the full-thickness skin graft donor sites will be dealt with in Chapter 4.

## When To Cut Skin With Scissors?

At The Johns Hopkins Hospital in the 1940s, it was common practice to disparage any surgeon who would deign to cut skin with scissors rather than a knife. "Sharp dissection techique" was the byword, and this was construed as condoning only the use of the scalpel in cutting or undermining skin. It was a point of pride not to be caught using the scissors for that type of dissection.

During those years, many of us had the opportunity of observing Alfred Blalock and his associates in cardiac surgery use the Metzenbaum scissors with great skill in dissecting out the structures of the mediastinum. Later, in Boston, I watched Frank Lahey use his knife to initially incise the epidermis and only about halfway through the dermis of the skin of the neck. He then completed the skin incision by cutting the remaining deep part of the dermis with curved scissors. The scalpel would not be used again during the operation and he would continue his thyroidectomies, using only the scissors to dissect all deep tissue planes—once beneath the upper dermal layer of the skin.

Although not as sharp as the edge of a scalpel, the blades of scissors have some special advantages in dissection. At times, they should even be used to cut skin! All surgeons should capitalize on these possibilities. By their very design, scissors produce a shearing and squeezing action on tissue. This action will close off and seal many small blood vessels that remain open and bleed if that same tissue is cut with a scalpel.

The slightly blunted tips of many surgical scissors also allow the surgeon to feel his way into proper fascial planes that are not as easily discovered if "knife-edge" sharp dissection is used.

When should skin be cut with the scissors? Very thin skin such as that of the eyelids, skin of the prepuce, or the vermilion of the lip is often more accurately and easily cut with scissors than with the knife.

Dr. Bradford Cannon has pointed out to the author that, if the scissors are drawn backward slightly in cutting thin skin, the motion will avoid producing a notch or scallop that may form in the skin if the scissors are pushed forward in the usual manner.

Thicker skin may often be cut most accurately by making the initial incision through the epidermis and most of dermis with a scalpel (Fig. 1.15A). The cut through the deep dermis and subcutaneous fat may then be completed with the scissors as popularized by Lahey (Fig. 1.15B). This not only reduces skin bleeding but allows a clean and accurate division of the deep skin edges. When curving or angled skin incisions are desired, this "knife-then-scissors" technique is especially helpful.

Chapter 2 will explore the use of scissors in cutting tissues other than skin.

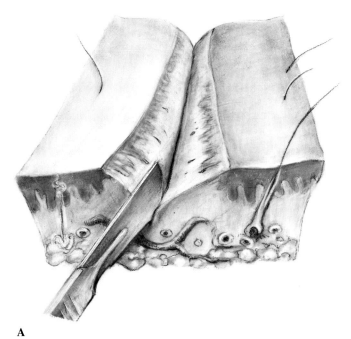

A

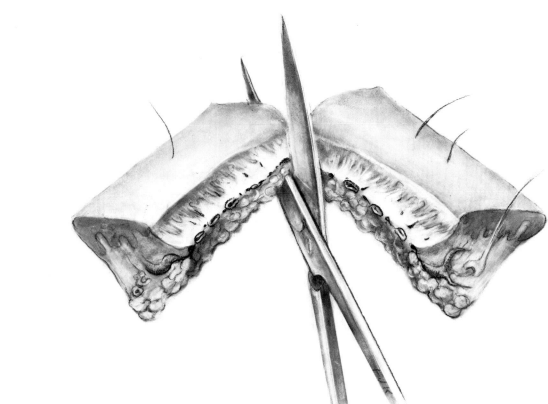

**Figure 1.15**                                    B

# 2
# Skills With Scissors

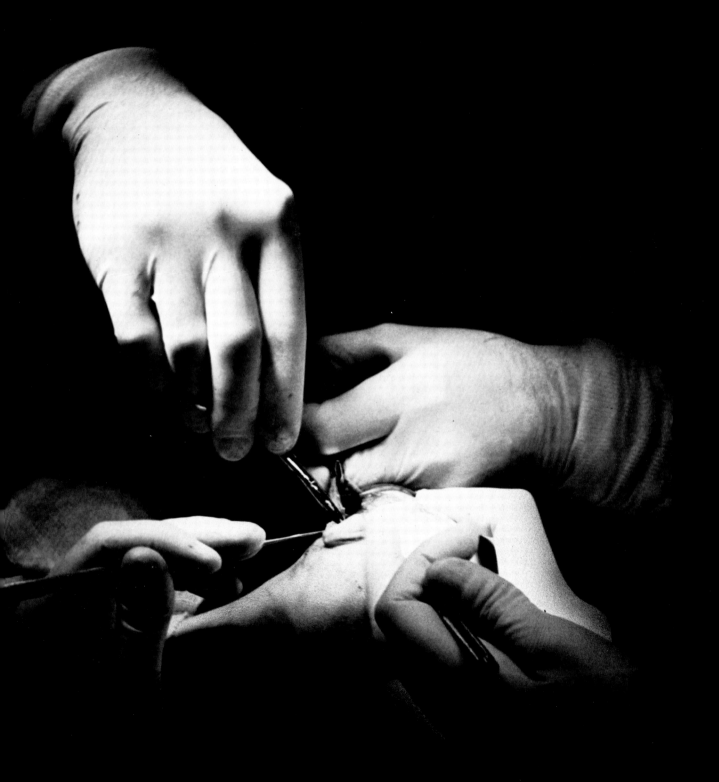

# 2

## Skills With Scissors

## Varieties of Scissors

Surgical scissors basically vary in only three major design features: (a) tips may be sharp or blunt, (b) blades may be curved or straight, and (c) handles may be long or short. There are many degrees of tip sharpness, blade curvature, and handle length, but different combinations of these three features account for the design and choice of use of almost all surgical scissors. Scissors with springs to open their blades or those with serrated edges to grasp tissue during cutting are designed for special purposes. The surgeon should analyze the task before him in selecting the right pair of scissors to do the job.

The typical pair of 6-inch-long scissors is designed and balanced for the normally sized adult human hand. Scissors handles should be longer than this only if the depth of a body cavity or surgical wound requires extra length of handle to reach the tissue conveniently.

Some scissors have very short handles (2 or 3 inches). They should be used only when the surgeon's hand will not enter a tiny space or when the scissors must be operated by holding the handle rings with the tips of the thumb and index finger. Even then, delicately tipped scissors with longer handles that fit the average human hand often do the job better than those with short handles. Delicate dissections are helped by small tips—not by small handles!

The sharpness or bluntness of scissor tips should be correlated with the density of tissue under dissection. When dissection is proceeding in scar tissue that is very dense, a sharp-pointed pair of scissors will be needed to penetrate between the collagen bundles. In Figure 2.1, the surgeon has encountered dense scar and thick palmar fascia in a patient with Dupuytren's

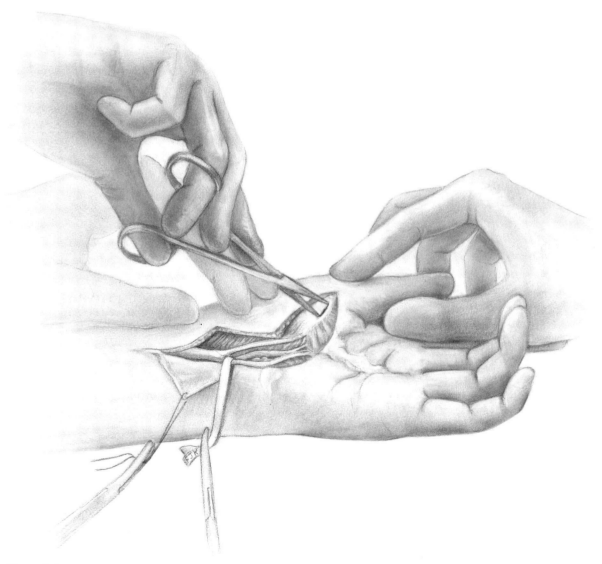

**Figure 2.1**

disease. He must remove it from the thenar eminence, but wishes to protect the motor nerve to the opponens muscle that lies just beneath. He has chosen a pair of sharp-tipped scissors that will penetrate the scar and then allow him to wedge open the scar as the points are separated. This opening is made parallel to the course of the motor nerve and is used to spot the nerve *before* cutting the underlying scar.

Note that the operator holds the scissors with his right index finger extended along the shaft, and that the thumb and ring fingers are pressed forward against the front of the finger rings. This allows him to exert force directly downward on the sharp tips and cause them to penetrate the scar. The fingers of the surgeon's left hand are placed on the thenar eminence so that the scissors may use them as a fulcrum to steady and direct the tips. The assistant surgeon's right hand

simultaneously fixes the patient's thumb to prevent any motion in the surgical field. A suture gently retracts a skin margin, and a piece of rubber tape protects and identifies branches of the median nerve that have already been dissected.

In other circumstances, when the surgeon is working in loose tissue planes that are free of old scar, slightly blunt-tipped scissors will provide both faster and safer dissections. Either the distinctly blunted tips of the Metzenbaum scissors or the slender but slightly rounded tips of the Jamieson scissors will serve admirably in almost all types of tissue dissection. Figure 2.2 shows a longer handled Metzenbaum and a shorter pair of Jamieson-handled scissors. Both are highly useful. The stout blades of curved Mayo scissors (not shown) may be needed in cutting through very heavily scarred tissues.

The use of scissors with slightly curved blades and tips gives versatility of approach angle and the ability to lift and palpate tissue to a degree not possible with straight-tipped scissors. Most good surgeons are instinctively aware of these advantages, and few will use a pair of straight scissors for routine dissections.

Straight-bladed scissors with either long or medium-length handles are, however, ideal for cutting the ends of sutures or ligatures. In these circumstances, the straight blades facilitate accurate and rapid positioning of the scissor tips just prior to cutting. Regardless of the scissor handle length, the speed and accuracy of cutting sutures will always be improved if the surgeon's assistant uses the index finger of his nondominant hand to brace the scissor tips against a fixed point on the patient. This finger acts as a fulcrum around which the scissors may be rotated to control exactly the level of the cut (Fig. 2.3).

The surgeon's assistant should never try to cut sutures with a single hand unless his second hand is occupied with a critical function that cannot be turned over to another member of the team. To do so will invite a trembling, unsteady scissor tip and a slower pace of surgery, and mark the assistant as an inexperienced amateur. The left hand should be used as a fulcrum to support the weight of the right hand as the latter quickly places, and then, closes the scissors. This will help relax the large muscles of the forearm. This relaxation in turn allows the small intrinsic muscles within the hand additional freedom to move the fingers rapidly into precise positions, to cut sutures quickly, and then to withdraw the scissors smoothly. The blades of the scissors should always be reopened

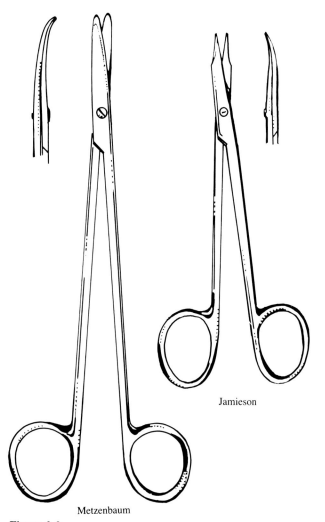

Jamieson

Metzenbaum

**Figure 2.2**

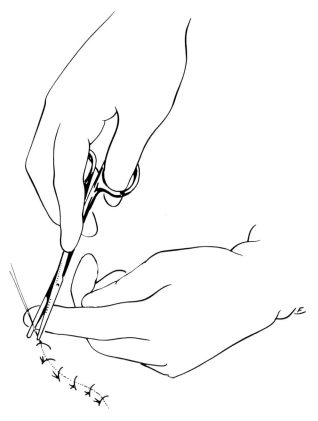

**Figure 2.3**

closing). Others have right-angled tips, or special curving handles (to reach around corners in deep holes). These unusual scissors are needed only occasionally, and the standard types (Fig. 2.2) will usually do most jobs quite nicely.

The young surgeon should strive to recognize when there are advantages that may accrue from the special features of any instrument, but in the absence of unusual anatomical conditions, he should select and use only those instruments that are most effective. Good surgery does not require a huge armamentarium of instruments. A selection of the most useful or indispensable instruments are described in the succeeding chapters.

## Holding the Scissors

### Fixation and Control Grips

Three points of fixation against the hand are needed for solid control of a pair of scissors. The standard and most useful grip is shown in Figure 2.4. The surgeon places his thumb and ring fingers of his right hand through the two finger rings of the scissors while the distal joints of the index and long fingers are curled beneath the shank. The index and long fingers thus provide stability and control the direction of thrust of the scissor tips. This grip works well when cutting tissue in a direction away from the surgeon's body or across the field from right to left (in the case of a right-handed surgeon). When one is using scissors with curved tips, the curve of the scissors should match the curve of the flexed fingers (i.e., the surgeon's palm should match the concave side of the scissor blades). This standard surgeon's grip is also

after cutting and before withdrawing the scissors. If this is not done, the closed blades may drag the ligature off a divided vessel and reinstitute significant bleeding. Thus, the assistant trains himself to (1) position the scissors, (2) close the blades, (3) open the blades, and (4) withdraw—in that order.

A few scissors have special designs such as double sharp edges (these will cut on both opening and

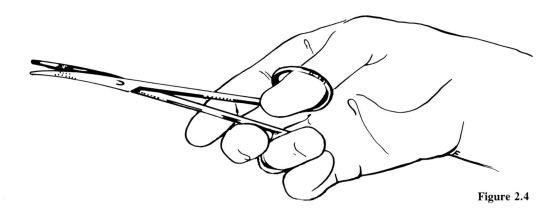

**Figure 2.4**

an excellent scissors grip for the assistant to use while cutting sutures with straight-bladed scissors.

### Position of Scissors Between Uses

Any assistant who is cutting sutures will find it convenient to learn the technique of flipping the tips of the scissors back into the palm of his hand between cuts. This is done as shown in Figure 2.5, by disengaging the thumb from the scissor ring as the scissors are rotated vertically and proximally with a flip of the index finger so that the tips come to rest alongside the assistant's wrist. The ring finger remains in the scissor ring. In this position, the ring and little fingers jointly clamp the scissors lightly but securely against the palm and wrist (Fig. 2.6). The scissor tips are now out of the way, and the assistant's thumb, index, and long fingers are free to handle the suction, to sponge, or to hold a retractor until the moment arrives to cut the next suture. At that point, the suction tip may be placed aside and the scissor tips may be swung smoothly back into position with a flexing of the little finger and a supination of the wrist. The thumb is again slipped into the second ring of the scissors and a cut of the suture is quickly made. This efficient

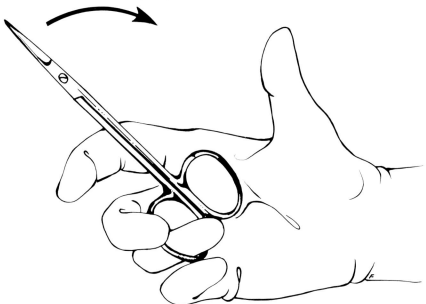

**Figure 2.5**

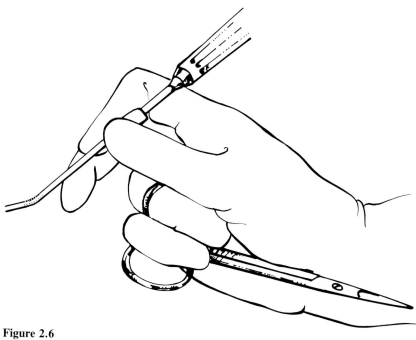

**Figure 2.6**

system for "tucking away" the scissors saves much wasted motion that would otherwise be required in repeatedly returning the suture scissors to the scrub nurse. At the same time, this system leaves both of the assistant's hands available for other duties.

### Tactile Control with Scissors

At times, the surgeon will find that tissue to be removed is extremely dense and that maximum stability of the scissors tips will be needed. In such cases, even greater control of the tips of the scissors is ob-

tained if the index finger is extended along the shanks directly behind the fulcrum of the scissors and the thumb tip is allowed to come through the ring and press down on one handle shaft. This allows the surgeon to produce downward pressure of the tips and blades against the tissue in the act of cutting. The ring finger and thumb remain placed through the scissor rings to give a wide base of support for the handle (Fig. 2.7). When using this grip, the surgeon may press the scissor tips strongly into and against dense fascia or scar, at the precise moment that the blades are closed.

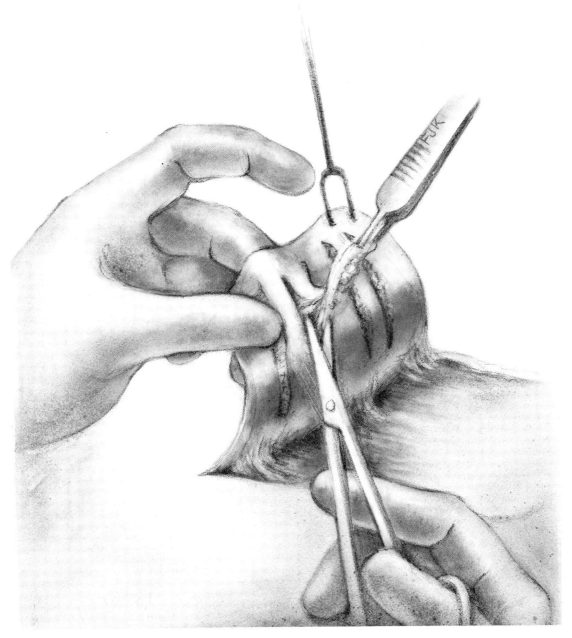

**Figure 2.7**

In Figure 2.7 the surgeon is removing dense scar from the deep surface of a previously elevated flap of skin. The scar on the flap has been incised down to the level of unscarred fat with several parallel strokes of the knife. The assistant is using a pair of forceps to lift one end of each strip of scar as the surgeon trims it away with Jamieson scissors. The extended index finger of his right hand (along the shaft of the scissors) helps him use the tips to press the sides of the scissor blades laterally as the right thumb pushes the tips down against the undersurface of the fat. These motions force the freed scar tissue to rise up between the opened blades and thus facilitate cutting. At the same time, the surgeon maintains exact tactile control by using the pulp and tip of his left long finger to assure himself that he is removing the scar at a uniform depth without damaging the important sub-dermal vascular plexus of the elevated flap of skin. The assistant is simultaneously using a two-pronged skin hook to gently stretch and flatten out the elevated flap, thus making scar removal more accurate and rapid.

In most operations, the deep surface of the skin will not already be scarred. In such circumstances, a pair of scissors with relatively blunt tips (e.g., Metzenbaum scissors) may be the most effective instrument. Whenever the surgeon dissects beneath skin with scissors, the curved tips are turned upward and may be palpated through the skin by the tip of the long finger of the operator's nondominant hand (Fig. 2.8). This bimanual palpation between the scissor tips and the pulp of the index finger on the skin surface allows identification of the exact depth of dissection. The method also reveals the density of any scar that may lie just beneath the skin, and helps the surgeon locate any intervening nodules of bone or soft tissue that may be of interest or require removal. Once the dissection has reached a point several inches from the skin incision, the surgeon may ask his assistant to exert traction on the skin margin with a sharp hook. This frees the surgeon's nondominant hand to move forward with the advancing scissor tips and continue with palpation of flap thickness.

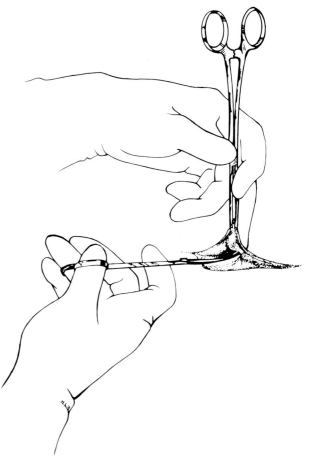

**Figure 2.8**

When working in loose fascia or along the sheaths of major blood vessels, the tips of the scissors may be fixed in a slightly separated position and then used to strip back and divide fascia along a linear path. This stripping action is shown in Figure 2.9 where it is being used to open the carotid sheath. The V-shaped opening between the tips remains set at a narrow angle, and the index finger can be used to guide the direction of dissection as the scissors are pushed forward. The technique should be used with caution if scar tissue is dense or if pathological tissue lies along the path of separation. This technique of stripping with the scissors is of great value to cardiothoracic surgeons.

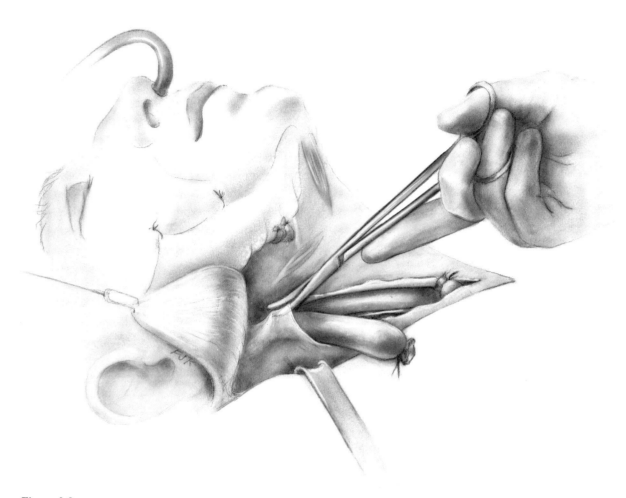

**Figure 2.9**

## Scissors Mechanics

### How the Hand Produces Shear Forces

When a surgeon uses a right-handed pair of scissors in his right hand, the scissor blades are closed by contraction of the adductor pollicis muscle while the muscles of thumb opposition simultaneously press thumb ring and handle of the scissors forward (away from the surgeon's palm). Simultaneously, the flexors of the long and index fingers assist the ring finger in pulling the finger ring and handle of the scissors back toward the palm. These opposing forces push the blades of the scissors into maximum proximity and increase the shear and cutting action of their edges. Whenever tissue is especially dense or tough, the need for this shear force increases. If this same (right-handed) pair of scissors is used in the left hand, these finger motions must be completely reversed to gain good shear action. As a result, right-handed surgeons have considerable difficulty in using scissors with their left hands. Most left-handed surgeons have used right-handed scissors since early childhood and manage to use them satisfactorily with either hand. For this reason, left-handed scissors are seldom needed, in modern operating rooms.

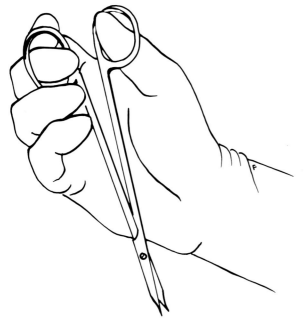

**Figure 2.10**

Another occasionally helpful grip when using the scissors is the reversed or "tips-toward-wrist" grip. Figure 2.10 shows that this position places the thumb and index fingers through the rings, but directs the tips and shaft of the scissors back along the palm of the hand and toward the ulnar side of the surgeon's wrist. The third point of stability in this grip is supplied by the ulnar border of the hand and the hypothenar eminence. The value of this grip lies in the fact that it enables the surgeon to cut directly back toward himself while maintaining full view of the working scissor tips. His scissor hand is curled behind the scissors and thus does not obstruct his vision. The second indication for use of this reversed grip is the cutting of tissue that lies under direct vision in a deep hole or cavity. In this circumstance, the tips of the scissors are allowed to fall away from the wrist and palm so that they may enter the cavity. The more standard grips of the scissors would force the surgeon to place his wrist in extreme pronation—motion that often places the back of his hand in a position that obstructs his own view of the operative field.

The above three basic scissor grips are those primarily needed for almost any type of surgery. Unusual grips that avoid placing the fingers inside the scissor rings, that use only two contact points for instrument control, or that artificially shorten the scissors length by backing up the handle within the palm are to be condemned. They usually represent a type of "stunting" and often delay the operation.

## Left-Handed Scissors

Left-handed scissors are available and are designed so that the shear forces on the blades may be produced by using the stronger muscles of the left hand on the scissors in exactly the same fashion as the fingers of the right hand are used in the control of right-handed scissors. However, as indicated earlier, left-hand surgeons (over 20% of current surgical residents) seldom bother to obtain left-handed scissors as they have learned how to develop excellent shearing action from right-handed scissors when using either hand. The reverse is not the case. The right-handed surgeon should avoid using his left hand to cut with scissors. The left-handed surgeon has this bimanual talent with scissors only because he has had much practice using right-handed scissors since early childhood (see section on "The Left-Handed Surgeon" in Chapter 8).

# When and How to Use Scissors in Surgery

## Functions of Scissors

Once the surgeon understands the mechanics and fundamental types of scissors, and has mastered the basic scissor grips, he should give some thought to the different functions of scissors in surgery. Scissors are used to (1) cut tissue and sutures, (2) spread and open tissue planes, (3) squeeze off and seal small blood vessels in the act of cutting, and (4) aid the surgeon in the palpation of tissue that comes to lie between his scissor tips and his fingertips.

The closed scissors may be swept from side to side and used as a tissue elevator and blunt dissector. This effectively extends the length of the surgeon's fingers and opens tissue planes when the vertical fascial attachments are not dense. If tissue density makes enlarging of a horizontal plane difficult, the inserted scissor tips may be spread to provide additional dissecting force. This will augment the side-to-side sweeping action of the closed tips.

## Using Scissors in Hilton's Maneuver

As the scissor tips are inserted into the tissue (Fig. 2.11A) and then opened (Fig. 2.11B), the blunted outer edges of the blades may encounter bands of attachment and blood vessels that need separation

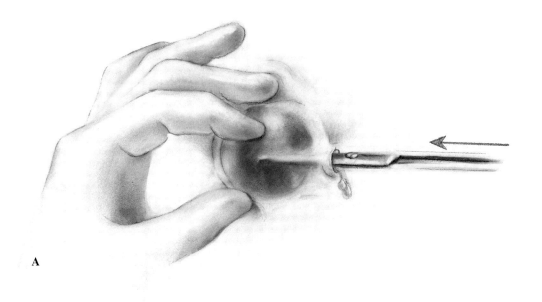

A

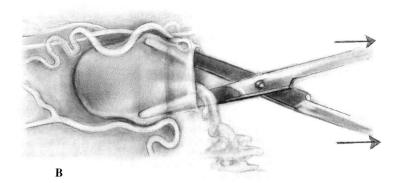

**Figure 2.11**

B

for good surgical exposure. When important nerves and major vessels transverse these septa, the closed scissors may first be tunnelled past these structures; the fully inserted blades are then opened widely; and the scissors withdrawn with the tips separated (Fig. 2.11*B*). The channel thus produced is often used to allow the escape of fluid or pus from a deep abscess, the center of which has first been penetrated by the closed tips. The surgeon may further enlarge this passage by inserting his finger, a drain, or another surgical instrument. This method makes use of the blunt outer edges of the opened scissor blades, on their withdrawal, to wedge apart the dense scar without using a sharp edge that would divide many adjacent nerves or vessels. This valuable scissors dissection technique was first described many years ago by Hilton and is known as Hilton's maneuver. Figure 2.12 shows its use in draining a large axillary abscess without injuring important nerves in the brachial plexus. *The sharp edges of the scissor blades are not used to open the tissues.* Double sharp-edged scissors should *not* be used in this fashion.

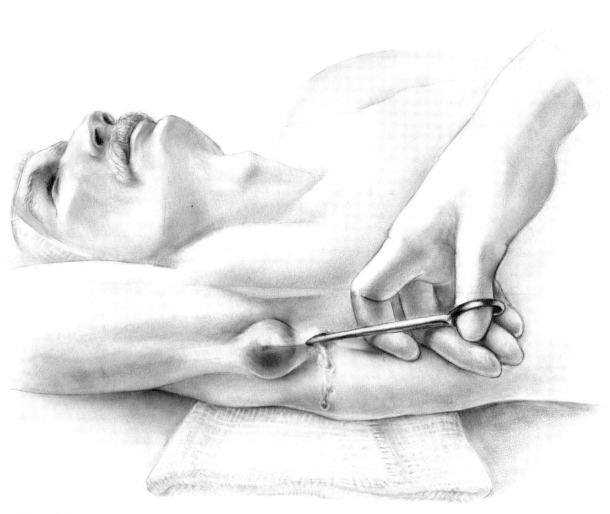

**Figure 2.12**

Thus, scissors may help the surgeon in several distinct and valuable ways: (1) They may be used as *shear cutters* to divide flaccid or fixed tissues or sutures. (2) They may be used as *push cutters* by opening the tips slightly and simply advancing the partly opened blades to strip tissues (Fig. 2.9). (3) The blunt sides of the blades may be used as lateral *sweep dis-* *sectors* or as *pull wedges* to spare nerves and vessels by withdrawing the opened scissors after first inserting them in closed position (Hilton's maneuver, Fig. 2.12). (4) They may be used to palpate the thickness and contents of elevated tissue, when aided by the operator's other hand as he feels the tissue between his finger and the moving scissor tips (Fig. 2.8).

# Cutting Sutures With Scissors

### Proper Length of Suture Ends

How much suture should be left beyond the knot in cutting sutures? In general, skin sutures that will require removal should be cut so as to leave the tails *as long as possible without leaving them so long that they will get entangled in the knot of the next suture to be tied.* When the ends of sutures are long enough to intermingle in tying (Fig. 2.13A), they become untied more easily, they collect and hold more crusts and clots, and later, they are more difficult to remove.

On the other hand, if sutures are cut shorter than they need to be (Fig. 2.13B), they will untie too easily (especially if there is regular cleaning of the suture line in the postoperative period), and they will be more difficult to grasp and elevate at the time of removal.

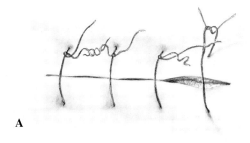

**A**

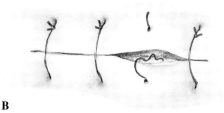

**B**

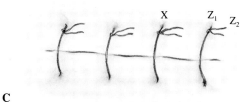

**C**

**Figure 2.13**

Most of us, when serving as surgical assistants, may have been tempted to ask the surgeon, "How do you want your sutures cut this morning? Too long or too short?" Any assistant should be able to watch the surgeon place his first skin suture and, without asking any questions, know the proper length to cut the ends of that first suture and any that follow.

If the surgeon is practicing sound mechanics, the width of the bite of the suture across the wound will tell the assistant exactly how far apart the subsequent sutures should be placed. In Figure 2.13C, the distance XY, or span of the suture, should usually approximate the distance $XZ_1$, or the distance between sutures. In turn, the suture ends should be cut short enough to avoid their becoming tangled in the next adjacent knot. The ends should not be so short as to make their removal difficult or allow them to become untied prematurely. This usually translates into desirable suture end lengths (indicated as the distance $Z_1Z_2$) that are 50% to 70% of the distance XY (the span between entrance and exit points of the needle across the suture line).

### Skin Sutures

Biomechanical studies show that small suture bites must be placed more closely together than large bites, to provide the same amount of approximation of the intervening skin margins. There are few mysteries about good techniques! Thus, if interrupted sutures are used to close an incision in very thin skin, the sutures will need to be both very close together and placed quite near the skin margins to avoid inversion or curling in of the edges. With thicker skin, the sutures may be placed further apart without loss in the quality of approximation. Do not forget that wide suture bites may leave wide permanent scars on the skin, especially if they are tied tightly or left in too long (see Chapter 6).

### Buried Sutures

Buried sutures are not subjected to as many frictional forces as are sutures on the surface of the body. Rubbing and movement tend to loosen the knots in skin sutures. Therefore, buried sutures may be cut with much shorter ends than skin sutures. Since buried sutures (except for pullouts) are not to be removed, the ends should only be long enough to prevent untying. Nonabsorbable sutures are usually cut just above the last throw of the knot; absorbable sutures are left with slightly longer (2 mm) ends. Absorbable sutures are somewhat stiffer and do have a greater tendency to become untied. Buried sutures (other than continuous nonabsorbable intradermal sutures that will be pulled out postoperatively) should probably never be placed so superficially in tissue that they engage the dermal layer of the skin. If either absorbable or nonabsorbable sutures are so placed, wound irregularities or suture extrusion will almost universally follow. Experimental evidence in human skin shows that buried intradermal sutures do not produce narrower ultimate scars than incisions closed with only skin sutures. This is true even when the wound closure has to be made under moderate tension.[1]

## Technique of Using Scissors to Cut Sutures

The surgical assistant must not depend on the scrub nurse to select his suture scissors. Many nursing programs still teach that "good" scissors should not be used to cut sutures for fear of dulling their edges. This hearkens back to several decades ago when coarse and heavy sutures were the rule. Today, the cutting of scar tissue and heavy fascia is infinitely more damaging to the sharp edges of scissors than is the cutting of relatively fine suture materials. The assistant should insist on a sharp pair of surgical scissors with handles of sufficient length to fit his hand and to reach easily to the depth of any cavities. A pair of scissors with straight, slightly blunted tips will give excellent directional control and are the scissors of choice, but scissors with slightly curved tips may also be used. The Metzenbaum scissors are too blunt-tipped to be ideal for cutting sutures in narrow spaces. By the same token, sharp-pointed scissors should be avoided as their tips may inadvertently injure important nearby structures as the scissors are being positioned for cutting.

When the assistant finds that he has been given a loose-jointed or dull-edged pair of suture scissors, he should politely but firmly pass them off the sterile field to the nurse and request that they be replaced and not used again unless repaired.

The most important single contribution that the assistant can make to the art of suture cutting is to anticipate the need and be ready. He should ready his

scissors when the surgeon starts to tie and move forward with his hands and the scissors (as a unit) just as the last knot is being tightened. The good surgeon will elevate both of the suture ends, holding them parallel to each other and inclined at such an angle that his own hands do not obstruct either his, or the assistant's, vision of the knot. The suture to be cut should be held in a plane that is at right angles to the line between the assistant's eye and the knot, as in Figure 2.14.

Note that the surgeon has retained the short end of the suture in his needle holder (he has just finished using it to make an instrument tie) and is holding the two ends of the suture together and quite still until after they are cut. He should freeze the motion of his hands as an unspoken signal to the assistant that he is ready for the suture to be cut. The assistant should be alert and poised to move in with scissors and both hands. Note that the ulnar border of his left hand is resting on the patient's forehead near the suture. His right hand rests the blades of his scissors on the radial border of his left index finger. The tips of the scissors are only slightly parted, the desired length of cut end is quickly estimated, and the scissors are closed, opened, and withdrawn. The sequence is never "close, withdraw, and open." If the scissors are not opened before withdrawal, the blades may cause a drag or tug on the suture. This is even more likely to occur if the scissors are dull.

At times, an assistant's second hand is engaged in an essential task (e.g., holding a critical retractor), and he finds himself with only a single hand available to cut sutures. In such circumstances, he should rest the hand holding the scissors against the patient before cutting. In all other circumstances, the nondominant hand is first placed on the wound edge or on some other stable point about 2 inches from the knot. The blades of the scissors are rested on this hand for stability and control (Fig. 2.14). This bimanual method allows the assistant to bring the scissors to the knot with speed and grace, even when it is necessary for him to fully extend his elbows to reach the cutting area. The scissor blades are opened only a few millimeters, and the tips are carefully watched to be sure that no tissue *beyond* the suture will be cut when they are closed. Although the movement of hands and scissors to the knot should be rapid, a brief reassuring pause and fine adjustment of the angle of the scissor tips before cutting the suture, is considered good form. Even the routine cutting of sutures can be done with style and professionalism!

[1]Winn HR, Jane JA, Rodeheaver GT, Edgerton MT, Edlich RF. Influence of subcuticular sutures on scar formation. Am J Surg 133:257–259, 1977.

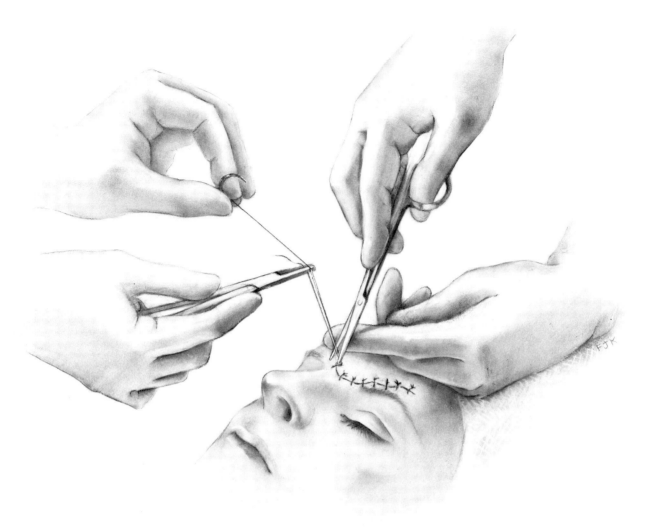

**Figure 2.14**

Sutures cannot be cut efficiently without a good view of the operating field. It is the surgical assistant's responsibility to anticipate the surgeon's hand positions and unobtrusively position himself so that he can see well when his moment arrives. It is not excusable for him to discover at the last moment that he is positioned so that he cannot see the operative field well enough to do his job.

When cutting sutures that will be left buried in the wound, the surgeon may request the cut to be "right on the knot." It is then appropriate to slide the slightly opened tips of the scissors down the suture ends until the last knot is felt as it bumps against one blade of the opened scissors. One blade of the scissor tips is then angulated or rotated upward about 45° above the last knot (leaving the other blade in contact

with the knot), and the suture is cut. If buried suture ends in subcutaneous tissue are left too long, they may function like unplanned drains and later extrude. Excessively long suture ends also increase the amount of nonliving material in the wound, thus adding to the inflammatory response.

### Cutting Moving Sutures

If sutures must be cut on tissue that is in motion, such as the beating heart or respiring lung, the assistant should reach over and take the long ends of the suture in his own nondominant hand before cutting. This will allow him to synchronize the up-and-down movements of suture and scissors with tissue movement at the moment of cutting. Even with non-moving sutures, whenever several in a row have been left long after tying and so that they may be cut all at one time, the assistant may again prefer to collect this row of sutures in his left hand, while cutting with the right.

### Cutting Steel

Cutting steel or other metallic sutures poses two special problems. Very fine steel wire may be cut with ordinary suture scissors without harm to the scissors. Larger caliber wire (sizes #30 and above) should be cut with wire cutters. The last knot (like all earlier knots) with wire should always be laid flat, and *the wire ends should not be lifted upward or be brought together for cutting.* Each end of the wire should be cut separately. This avoids the looping and loss of effectiveness of the last knot. It is also important that steel wire ends be secured in a clamp or fingers before they are cut free. This avoids having them jump into the wound or someone's eye when cut.

## Use of Scissors in Combination with Other Instruments

The right-handed surgeon will often use his left hand to retract tissues or palpate through the skin at the same time that he is using the scissors in his right hand (Fig. 2.8). This ability to feel with the scissors allows safe and rapid, blunt or sharp dissection in areas where tissue plane attachments are less dense than in adjacent structures. To use this method safely, the surgeon must know his regional anatomy with great accuracy. This technique improves greatly with practice.

### Bimanual Techniques

Surgery at its best is always a two-handed profession, and the surgeon must often use a forceps, retractor, suction tip, elevator, or other instrument in his left hand, in coordination with use of the scissors in his right. Such bimanual skills greatly increase the range of actions that may be accomplished with the scissors. For example, the surgeon may retract the edge of a skin incision with a sharp hook held between the thumb and index finger of his left hand. As he dissects beneath the skin with the scissors, he may appear to be working blindly, but he is able to maintain an exact depth of dissection by palpating the scissors through the skin with the pulps of his left long, ring, and little fingers (Fig. 2.8). By maintaining proper direction of the countertraction on the skin edge with the hook, he avoids buttonholing the skin or dissecting too deeply. This also prevents important deep structures from becoming so flaccid that they are inadvertently dragged upward with the elevated skin and caught between the closing blades of the scissors (see Chapter 4).

### Ambidexterity

Such combinations of instrument use by both hands of the surgeon have multiple ramifications that will be enlarged on in later chapters. There are many occasions when the shape, angle, or depth of a wound makes it prudent for the surgeon to shift his scalpel or scissors to his nondominant hand and use his forceps or another instrument in the dominant hand. A little practice makes these movements surprisingly easy. All good surgeons develop a degree of ambidexterity in using each common instrument.

# 3
## How to Hold Skin

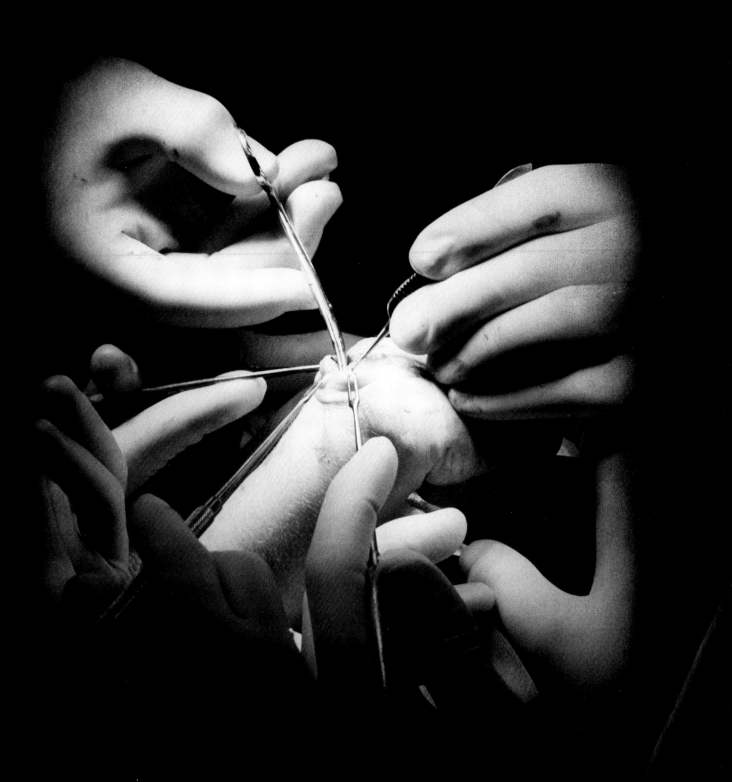

# 3
## How to Hold Skin

*God heals wounds—I only dress them.*
Ambroïse Paré, 1555 A.D.

Skin, like all other tissue encountered in surgery, should be held as gently as possible. Once incised, it should be lifted, retracted, repositioned, and resutured with as little disturbance as possible to its homeostatic mechanisms.

Whenever we upset normal physiology, we damage the patient's mechanisms of wound healing. All trauma is injurious to cells! Each injured cell will place added demands on the body's recovery mechanisms. This adds stress and reduces the patient's state of health.

## Instruments Used to Hold Tissue

### Fingers

America's first full-time plastic surgeon was Baltimore's John Staige Davis. As a student at The Johns Hopkins School of Medicine in the 1940s, the author had the privilege of watching this remarkable pioneer work in the operating room.

He was a tall and almost gangling surgeon with long fingers and large hands. He would often place the head of a small infant in his lap while repairing a cleft of the lip. He would use sutures that his nurse would prepare from long strands of hair he had personally selected from the tail of a favorite horse. At times he would seem to ignore the shiny surgical instruments on his Mayo stand as he seemed almost to fumble with the tiny tissues of that baby's lip. To the uninitiated his large fingers would have seemed awkward in handling such small structures.

Being new to the world of surgery, I wondered why Dr. Davis didn't elect to use those interesting sharp and special tools to make the operation look ''more elegant.'' The answer lay in observing the way Dr. Davis' wounds healed. In the days after surgery, it was obvious that the suture lines in those babys' lips healed with little evidence of scar or reaction to the surgery. It was years before I appreciated how important the soft touch of those gentle fingers had been to that healing. The repair of those wounds was much improved by Dr. Davis' restraint and his minimal use of instruments with sharp tips that crush, tear, cut, or otherwise damage living cells. Dr. Davis knew that *fingers are the best and gentlest of all surgical instruments,* and he used them whenever they would do the job.

This use of the fingers to hold skin is illustrated in Figure 3.1. The surgeon has already placed his suture needle through both sides of the skin incision. He is using the thumb and index finger of his left hand as his only instruments to fix the skin margin as the needle tip engaged and then penetrated the skin on the emerging side of the incision. This produces minimal cell damage. Holding the skin edge with toothed forceps would have been less kind.

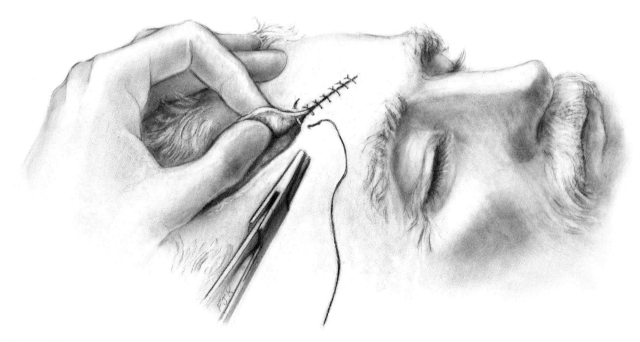

**Figure 3.1**

Later Staige Davis showed me another method of fixing the mobile edge of a skin incision, using a folded sponge to brace the loose edge of skin as he pushed the needle point through the skin and up into the sponge. Figure 3.2A shows how several layers of sponge may be used to brace a skin margin as the needle engages it. In placing a suture through the skin on the first (needle-entering) side of the incision, the point of the needle is simply directed downward at right angles to the skin surface, and the resistance of the underlying tissue is used to fix the skin as the needle penetrates. On the second (needle-emerging) side, the operator places the needle tip at the precise point on the underside of the skin. He then covers the skin with the sponge, taking care to separate two fingertips at the approximate point of emergence of the needle. He next advances the needle with the needle holder so that the needle tip emerges through the skin and enters the sponge as he continues to press the sponge and skin down firmly.

The sponge is then lifted (Fig. 3.2B) to expose the needle tip, which is then grasped by the needle holder and withdrawn. This method of placing sutures avoids injuring the skin with any instrument other than the tip of the needle. The technique allows accurate placement of the suture—even quite close to the cut margin of the skin.

In using this method to close a skin incision, the tip of the needle is placed under the skin edge to engage a small amount of the deep dermis. Pressure on the sponge is then applied in a manner that will roll the skin backward (away from the wound margin) and evert the edge modestly before the needle is pressed upward and out through the remaining thickness of the skin. The tip of the needle should enter the sponge midway between the surgeon's thumb and index fingertips. This simple maneuver has served me well on the "emerging" side of suturing incisions for many years. It is of particular usefulness when the skin to be sutured has a very thin dermal layer.

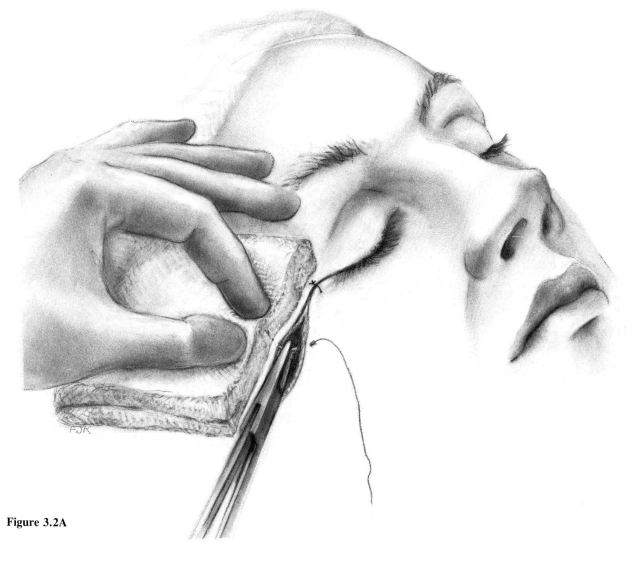

**Figure 3.2A**

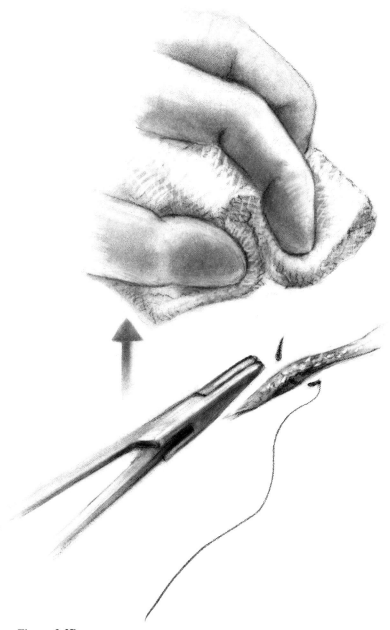

**Figure 3.2B**

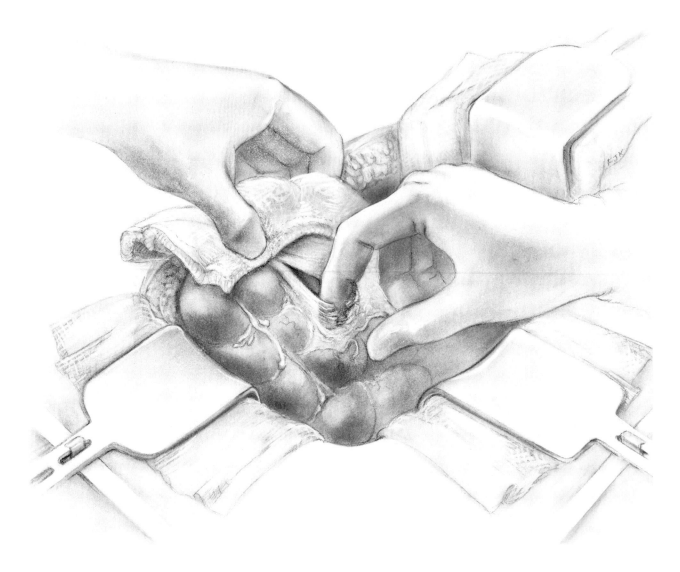

**Figure 3.3**

The hands and fingers may also be used to gently lift the margins of wounds in order to place retractors, introduce packs, allow irrigation, or simply to aid the surgeon with the introduction of his opposite hand for better palpation.

The gloved hand always should be moist and free of any irritating glove powder before contacting opened tissues. If these two simple precautions are followed, it is almost impossible to do damage to the tissues by holding them with ''the surgeon's ten best instruments''—his fingers. No other surgical tool has the ability to convey maximal tactile sensations to the surgeon. The temperature, density, flexibility, thickness, and consistency of the tissue will all be registered by the holding hand. The use of a thin surgical glove will maximize these tactile capabilities.

Adhesions that have formed between loops of bowel or lobes of the lung are readily separated by the surgeon's index finger. This dissecting finger tells him instantly when the resistance reaches a point that spells danger of tearing or penetrating a viscus if he pushes any harder. In Figure 3.3, the surgeon is using his index finger to break up adhesions and free up loops of bowel. The sensitivity of his fingertip will immediately tell him when he reaches adhesions that are so dense that continued blunt finger dissection would risk tearing the delicate walls of the intestines. Here he is using a moist gauze pad in his left hand to prevent it from slipping as he exerts counter traction to assist the dissecting finger.

The wound margins in Figure 3.3 are held by self-retaining retractors. Whenever such fixed retractors are used, they should be placed over moist gauze pads to protect the wound margins, as shown. The blades should be tightened just enough for adequate exposure, and they should be released at intervals (15 to 20 minutes) during long operations so as to allow circulation to return and perfuse the tissues beneath each blade.

### Skin Hooks

Contrary to popular belief, the sharp skin hook and sharp deep tissue hook are not modern instruments. These important tools were used over 2,000 years ago, and beautifully crafted surgical hooks have been recovered from the surgical clinic that was buried at Pompeii in 79 A.D. (Fig. 3.4).

Next to the human finger, these simple curved metal points at the end of a handle offer the gentlest technique for lifting or retracting tissue. The hook points should be quite sharp and should not be curved back on themselves beyond 180° with the long axis of its handle or they will be difficult to disengage from tissue. The handle of such a hook should be only 4 to 5 inches in length unless retraction is needed in a very deep cavity.

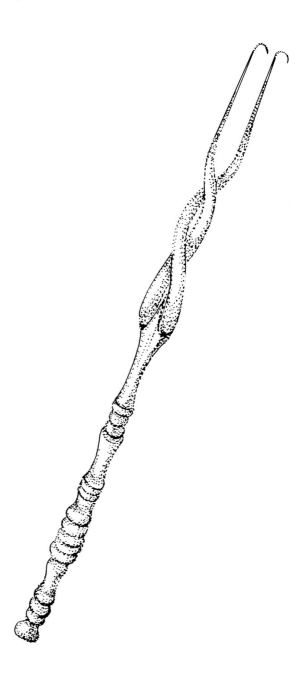

**Figure 3.4**

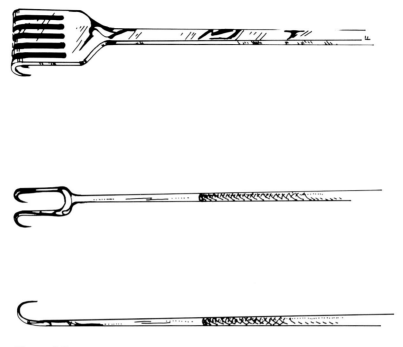

**Figure 3.5**

Hooks may be single, double, or multiple (Fig. 3.5). A tool with three or more points is called a "sharp rake" or "cat's paw" retractor. It is used when a very wide expanse of skin or a wide section of body wall or cavity needs retraction in a single direction.

It is usually wise to set sharp hook tips firmly into the tissue with definitive finger pressure, as the first step of retracting. When these tips are fixed securely in position, they will allow the assistant to lift the tissue in one of several different vectors without slipping of the retractor. The length of the handle allows the assistant's hand to be out of the way and well back from the margin of the wound.

If the points of a skin hook have become somewhat dull, the assistant or surgeon should take special pains to set the tip by pressing it into a new area of tissue whenever the hook needs to be repositioned.

In Figure 3.6 the surgeon is using his right hand to suspend the double skin hook over the edge of the skin he wishes to retract. He then uses the thumb and index finger of his nondominant hand to set the points of the hook firmly in the tissue. He pinches the hook tips and tissue together until he feels them engage.

Once the hook is set, he slides the dominant hand upward to hold the hook handle and clamps the hook tips into position with the long finger of that hand as shown in Figure 3.7. By these simple motions, he has gained excellent and secure control of the wound margin. He may then elevate, undermine, advance, or suture with great ease and with minimal trauma to the retracted tissue. As dissection proceeds he may choose to release and reset the hook at a deeper point beneath the margin to improve exposure or tissue traction.

Hooks should *not* be used to retract bowel, lung, liver, or other soft tissues that would be likely to bleed, tear, or be perforated.

## Forceps

Forceps are made with smooth jaws or with small, sharp, interlocking teeth. When smooth-jawed forceps are used, more force or tissue compression is required to lift tissue against resistance without slipping. Thus, it is easier on tissue if it is handled with toothed forceps whenever possible. The damage from toothed jaws may be further dispersed if many fine

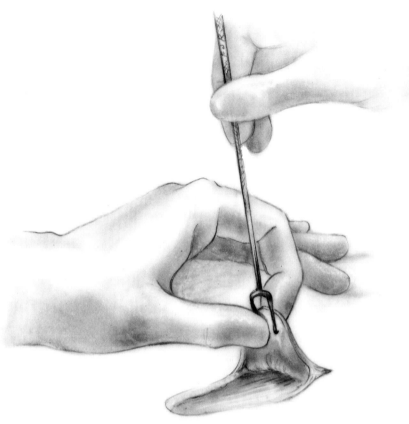

**Figure 3.6**

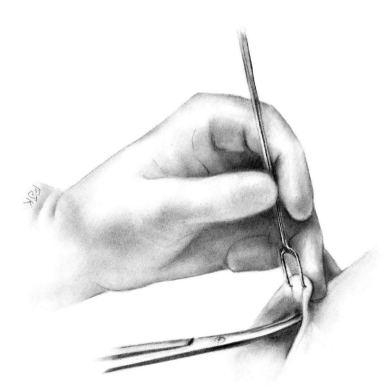

**Figure 3.7**

teeth line the jaws rather than three to five larger ones. Even a mouse-tooth forceps that contain only three teeth will crush many living cells each time its jaws are used to pick up and compress tissue with sufficient force to allow cutting or retracting. Surgeons interested in protecting tissue find that a skin hook has advantages over use of the toothed tissue forceps in many surgical maneuvers.

Smooth-jawed forceps should be used in two circumstances:

1. If the tissue to be grasped is likely to be damaged or torn by toothed forceps (for example, a thin-walled vein or lymphatic);
2. When the teeth of toothed forceps would get entangled in the tissue or material being handled (for example, in packing gauze into a cavity).

The most useful types of forceps are shown in Figure 3.8. On the left is the three-toothed Adson forceps. This is widely useful in surgery. The surgeon must school himself to pinch the jaws together with only the minimum force required to do the job. If he notes deep tooth indentations or "footprints" in the skin after removing the forceps, he can be sure he has killed many cells. The smooth-jawed forceps are shown in the center. They are of value in lifting thin-walled veins or in placing packs or drains. The small Wainstock-type forceps on the right are quite fine-tipped and thus useful in picking up tiny blood vessels for electrodessication. Their short handles may sometimes be bothersome, especially if they are used in deep holes but longer handles will make the long delicate tips somewhat unstable. The multitoothed Brown-Adson forceps shown at the bottom of the figure provide wider areas of fixation and are of value when larger bites of tissue need to be fixed or moved with significant force or in grasping slippery materials such as cartilage or surgical implants.

*All good forceps should have very light springs to open their jaws.* When the spring is strong, the surgeon is unable to appreciate exactly how firmly he is grasping the tissue. In addition, the strong spring will soon tire the small intrinsic muscles (lumbricals, interossei, adductor pollicis, and flexor pollicis brevis muscles) in the surgeon's hand, thus reducing the skill and ease of his movements.

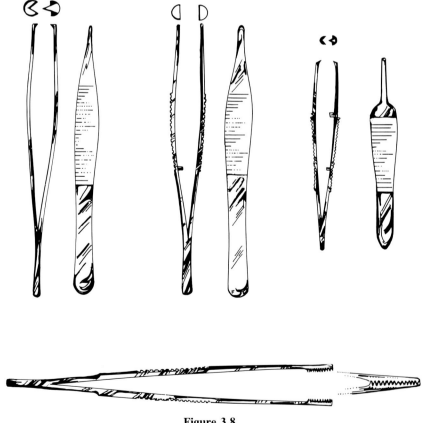

Figure 3.8

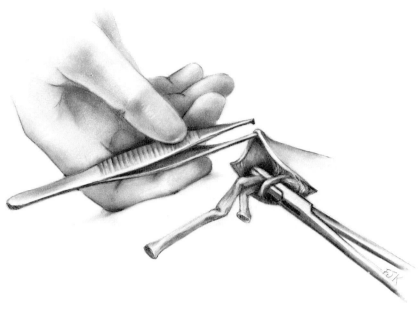

**Figure 3.9**

The experienced surgeon will learn to use toothed forceps in a way that reproduces many of the atraumatic features of sharp skin hooks. Figure 3.9 shows how he may lift the skin by pressing firmly against the tissue with a single jaw (the "lifting jaw") of the forceps, while at the same time he applies little or no pressure to the top (or "down-pressing") jaw of the forceps. This maneuver uses the hooklike action of the tooth or teeth in one jaw of the forceps to retract the tissue while avoiding the damaging effects of tissue crush produced by more conventional use of equal pressure on both jaws of the forceps. Once an instinct for handling tissues in a kindly fashion has been de-veloped, the surgeon will unconsciously employ this differential pressure method of using his forceps whenever it is practical. The surgeon may also reduce damage from the use of forceps by carefully selecting the tissue he grasps. Some tissues are much more sensitive to crushing forces than others. Figure 3.10A shows the way many surgeons pick up skin with forceps. With this technique, the teeth damage the epidermal cells and may even leave permanent surface scars. If instead the skin is picked up by grasping the fascia or relatively acellular dermis just beneath the surface (Fig. 3.10B), the damage is less and the better eversion of the margin will often assist in the placing of sutures or other surgical maneuvers.

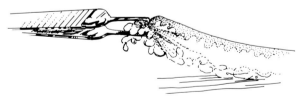

**Figure 3.10A**

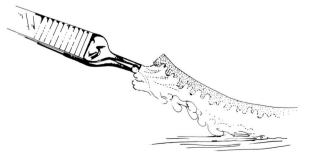

**Figure 3.10B**

## Retractors

In speaking of operations, the late Glover Copher of St. Louis often said, "They are all easy if you can see them." By that he meant to stress that excellent surgical exposure adds greatly to the safety and ease of surgery.

By the same token, the retraction of skin and wound margins and the displacement of internal solid and hollow viscera are made much easier if the surgeon starts out by making his incision in the proper location and of adequate dimensions. *The best assistant in the world will have retractor problems if the incision is inadequate.* Surgeons should remember that, after healing, *patients are far less troubled about the length of an incision than they are about its width and contour irregularities!*

### Types of retractors

The choice of the appropriate retractor makes surgery a joy. Retractors may be smooth or sharp, wide or narrow, stiff or flexible, self-retaining or handheld.

They may also have special features such as winches that will force open a rib cage or fiberoptic lights may be mounted on their blades to illuminate deep cavities. Some may have special shapes to fit into the vagina or to lift the lobes of the liver during gallbladder surgery. Others are designed to control tongue position while at the same time, they hold open the jaws and provide a groove for an endotracheal airway. The Dott-Dingman mouth gag shown in Figure 3.11 is of great value in operating within the oral cavity or oropharynx under general anesthesia. The tongue and lower jaw are pushed in a caudad direction and the mouth is opened as the ratchet on the tongue blade is tightened. Two double-pronged sliding hooks are set on the upper teeth or alveolar ridge so as to avoid pinching the upper lip against the teeth. Two adjustable side arms may be set to retract the corners of the mouth laterally. Several sizes of tongue blades are available for patients of different ages. The groove

in the tongue blade centers the endotracheal tube and helps prevent its displacement. Like all self-retaining retractors it should be placed carefully and released at intervals to avoid tissue injury.

All good retractors are designed to give the surgeon sufficient exposure of his operative field so that he may have optimum vision and working room. This must be done so as to produce the least additional damage to adjacent normal organs and to the margins of the surgical wound.

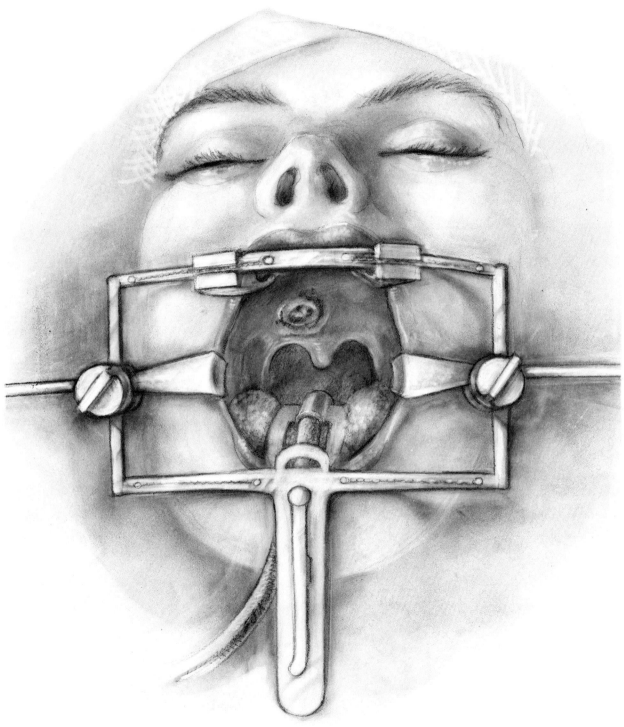

**Figure 3.11**

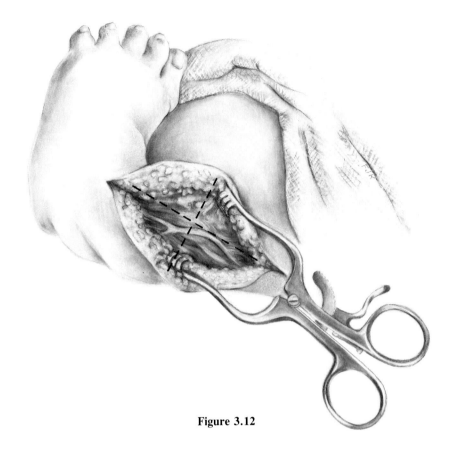

**Figure 3.12**

Self-Retaining Retractors

Self-retaining retractors have the advantage of saving the back and arm muscles of a surgical assistant, but they also have certain disadvantages.

The fixed position of a self-retaining retractor will often arrest the circulation in the stretched tissues about the incision. If this is continued for long, it may result in venous thrombosis, nerve damage, or even ischemic gangrene. The surgeon must take care to avoid excessive stretching of the tissues, and he should release the retractor at reasonable intervals to allow reperfusion of the ischemic areas. In Figure 3.12 a locking device on the retractor handle maintains the spread of this self-retaining device as the surgeon works on a congenitally deformed leg with a severe clubfoot.

Some self-retaining retractors are held in place by spring-loading mechanisms rather than locking devices. These are gentler on tissues, but they too should be repositioned at intervals in long operations.

Handheld Retractors

The hands of a thinking, restless, fatigable human being on the handle of most retractors give great advantages to the use of handheld retractors as compared to the self-retained variety.

The alert assistant holding a retractor will instinctively vary the position of its blade and handle to let the maximum amount of light into a wound. He will pull harder (even without a request!) if he sees that the surgeon briefly needs a little extra room to work. He will automatically ease up his pressure on the tissues when the surgeon is working in a more remote part of the surgical field. Whenever fatigue requires him to rest the muscles of his own hand and arm, the tissue beneath the blade of his retractor will also get a much-needed flow of oxygen and nutrients to its capillary network.

In plastic surgery, as well as in other specialties, the blood supply of vital tissue is often marginal. It is wise for all surgeons to develop special routines to minimize retraction injury. One such routine is the simple habit of holding one's breath during the period that a retractor is either compressing a vital structure such as the common carotid artery or occluding the flow through the pedicle of a flap of skin or muscle. When the breath-holding surgeon begins to experience air hunger himself (after 2 to 3 minutes), he auto-

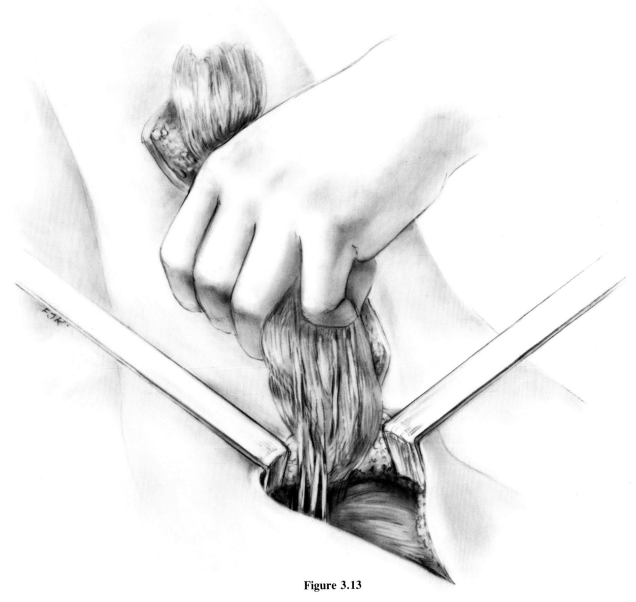

**Figure 3.13**

matically pauses in his dissection, takes a breath, and simultaneously releases the retractor so that the tissues may also gain relief. Flaps with significantly reduced circulation may infarct and die when retraction is not intermittently released. Flaps of similar design have been shown experimentally to survive when this simple routine is employed.

In Figure 3.13 the manual traction on the muscle and the resulting tension that is being exerted on the freed-up vessels in the pedicle of this latissimus dorsi musculocutaneous flap are stopping blood flow. If this pull on these vessels is excessive, or is continued too long, muscle necrosis will result. If the surgeon and assistant have the simple habit of breath holding in such circumstances, there is little danger of either excessively prolonging this period of flap ischemia, as

the traction on the muscle and vessels will be released after short intervals.

The surgical assistant should remember that hooked or sharp-pointed retractors allow better blood flow through elevated tissues than do flat and smooth-bladed retractors.

Flat retractors may also cause damage if their blades are turned or angled so that their edges cut into soft tissue such as a lobe of the liver or the spleen. In Figure 3.13 the right-angled retractors are properly inclined so as to retract the skin margins with minimal injury. Much of the danger of a malpositioned retractor will be avoided if a moist wet pack or sponge is draped over a wound margin before placing the metal blade in position (Fig. 3.3). This wet pad also reduces drying out of the tissues along the wound margins.

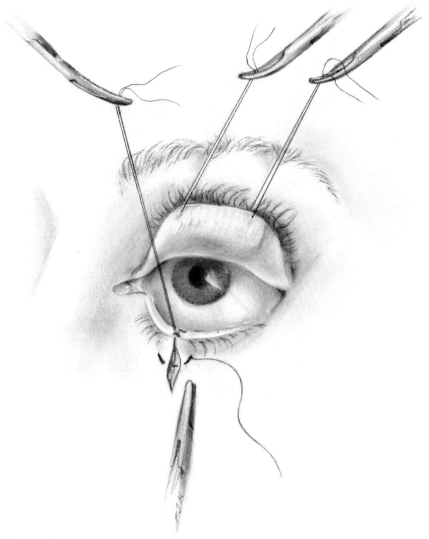

**Figure 3.14**

Suture Retraction

Sutures may serve as retractors if their ends are left long. As in Figure 3.14, they are particularly helpful in fixing or everting small mobile structures such as the inner surface of the eyelid while additional sutures are placed to complete the closure of a defect in the lower eyelid. Suture retraction should always be considered when delicate structures are going to require intermittent retraction and release over a period of time. A word of warning: If clamps are placed on the ends of retraction sutures, they should not be left unattended (i.e., unheld). To do so invites the risk of having someone pick up the clamp, and not realizing that its jaws are clamped on the suture, suddenly tear the suture from the tissue.

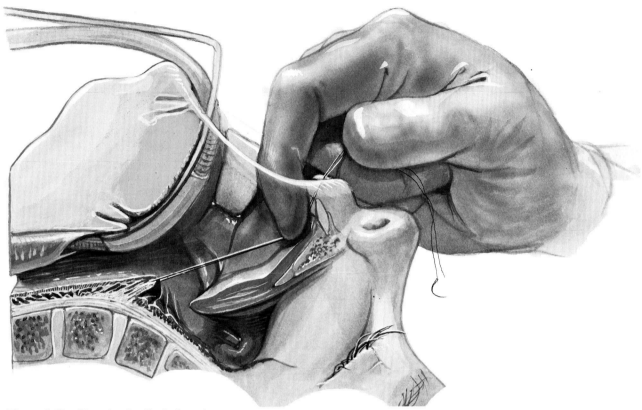

**Figure 3.15   (Drawing by Craig Luce.)**

Some traction sutures may be placed so as to drag inaccessible tissue into view in deep recesses which would not allow the introduction of other types of retractors. An example of this principle is seen with surgery on the posterior wall of the laryngopharynx. The posterior pharyngeal constrictor muscles and mucosal surface may be advanced cephalad several inches by traction on sutures placed in appropriate areas. In Figure 3.15, the surgeon has placed his first traction suture through the mucosa and the superior constrictor muscle at the midline of the pharynx. He is using the index finger of the right hand to push the suture up against the roof of the mouth and thus slide the mobile pharyngeal wall in a cephalad direction. This, in turn, allows him to place his next suture in the posterior pharynx at a point about 2 cm more caudad in the pharynx. He then elevates the tissues further by traction on this second suture until he has placed enough sutures to retract the tissues sufficiently to visualize and carry out needed surgical maneuvers in the posterior pharynx. Such retraction and exposure in the back of the pharynx is virtually impossible with any type of retractor other than sutures.

### Retraction with tissue crushing instruments

At times tissues that are necrotic or pathological may need to be retracted during dissection. In such cases, since these tissues are destined for removal during the course of the operation, the use of a tenaculum, towel clip, or Kocher clamp may offer the most practical and efficient handle for retraction. The Kocher clamp shown in Figure 3.16 has strong jaws and a secure handle lock. In Figure 3.17 it is being used to provide a secure grasp on a gallbladder that is being removed. No crushing clamp should be used on tissue that will be left in the body and expected to heal.

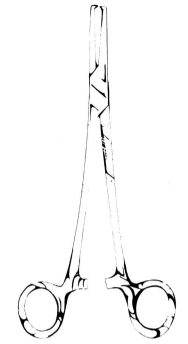

**Figure 3.16**

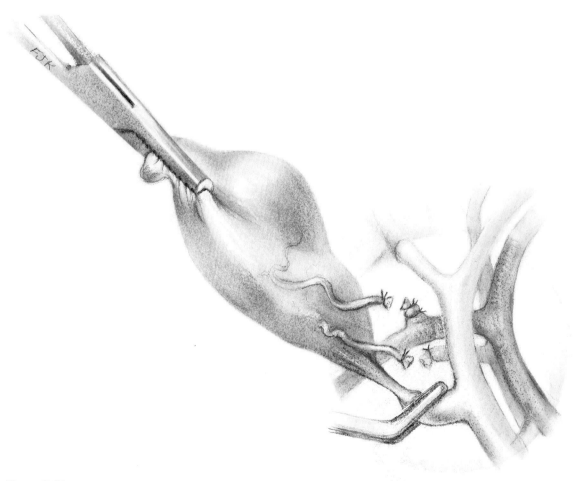

**Figure 3.17**

## The Surgical Assistant's Role

The surgical assistant should observe a simple and practical protocol if he is to offer optimum help with wound retraction. If exposure is poor, the first assistant should make it his business to find the first practical moment and method to provide it. This may be accomplished by a simple repositioning of the retractors held by the second assistant, or it may involve a courteous suggestion to the surgeon that the wound be repacked or that the incision be extended.

## The Moving Wound Principle

One method of improving surgical exposure without enlargement of the incision is to use retractors to shift a mobile skin opening to and fro to reveal different parts of the deep surgical field. This method is particularly applicable in those parts of the body where the skin and subcutaneous tissue are quite movable over the underlying structures.

In Figures 3.18 and 3.19, the principle of the "moving wound" to increase exposure is used to re-

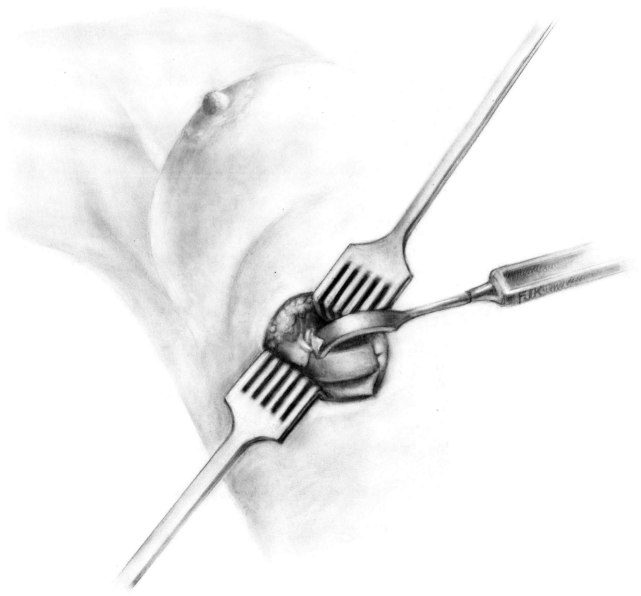

**Figure 3.18**

move a long (16 cm) segment of rib (for bone grafting) through a short (5 cm) skin incision. The incision is first drawn anteriorly and inferiorly by two rake retractors (Fig. 3.18) to start the elevation of the periosteum from the rib with a sharp elevator. The rakes are then replaced by deeper bladed blunt retractors, the opening in the skin of the chest is then retracted upward and toward the axilla, exposing the lateral and posterior parts of the rib (Fig. 3.19). The elevation of the periosteum is completed, and an angled bone cutter has been inserted in preparation for division of the rib at a point 10 cm behind the posterior end of the original skin incision. The coordinated movement of the retractors by an alert assistant makes the moving wound principle seem quite natural and easy.

If an operation is going slowly or encountering difficulties, in most instances it will be improved by better visualization of the operative field. Better adjustment of the overhead lights may frequently be needed.

The first assistant has a responsibility to assess the exposure and overall conduct of the operation. *He should spare the surgeon from mechanical supporting activities as much as his experience and imagination will allow.*

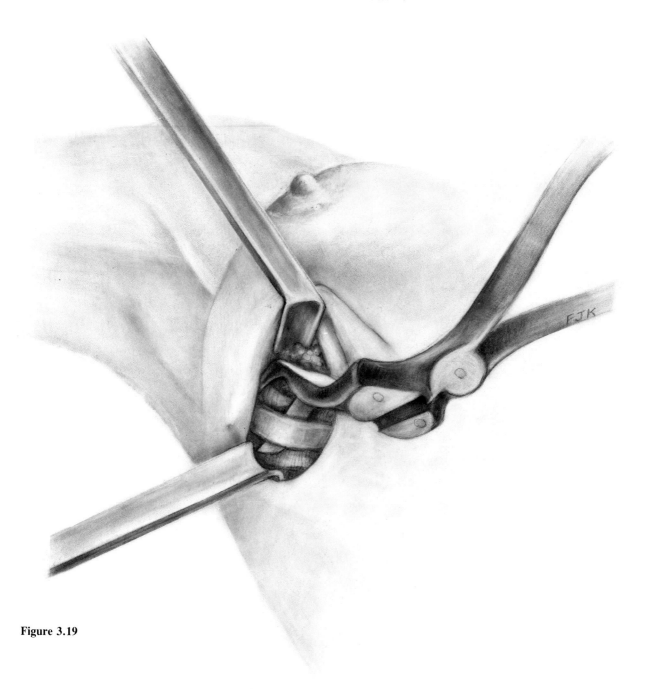

**Figure 3.19**

# 4

## Dissection and
## Skin Undermining

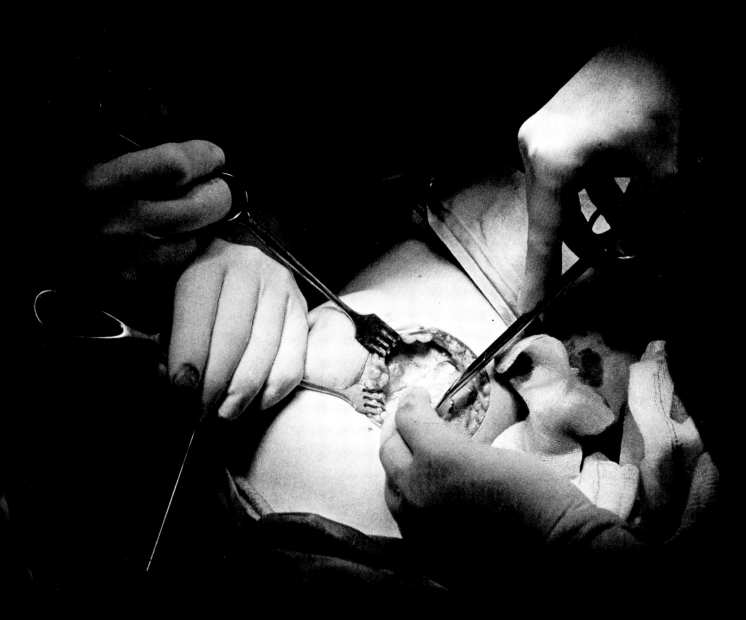

# 4

## Dissection and Skin Undermining

## Which Instrument to Use?

### Fingertip Dissection

Living tissue planes should be opened with the smoothest and bluntest instrument that will do the job without the need for excessive force. If the surgeon is required to apply heavy pressure on his instrument in order to open and separate tissue, there is danger that nerves, blood vessels, and other structures may be torn, with resultant bleeding, loss of exposure, and delayed healing.

The surgeon's index finger will readily dissect many lightly adherent normal tissue planes, and at times will safely open even avascular layers of col-

lagen bundles that have formed at the sites of old scars. In the act of such a dissection, the fingertip will often detect larger vessels or nerves that transverse these tissue planes from deep to more superficial positions. The discovery of these structures by palpation allows clamping, cutting, and cauterization with minimal blood loss. If the dissecting finger is used in combination with the pulp of the thumb, the surgeon will gain a bidigital quality from his palpation. The thickness, density, and temperature of tissue may be accurately assessed by holding it between the pulp of of the thumb tip, resting on the skin surface and the pulp of the index fingertip, within the wound. This type of bidigital dissection and palpation is illustrated in Figure 4.1. The surgeon is using his index finger to

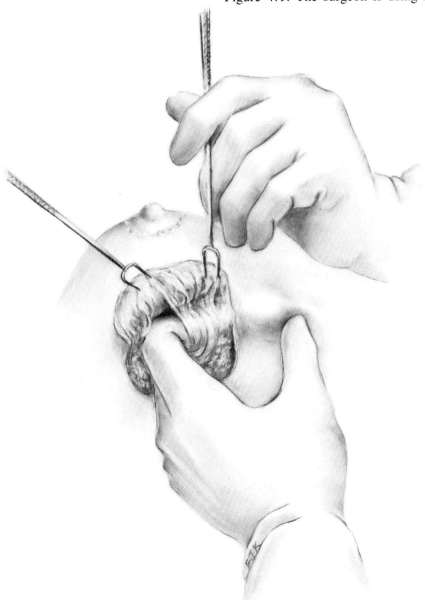

**Figure 4.1**

separate the tissues in the lateral aspect of the breast. The tip of this finger has encountered a firm nodule. At that point the surgeon brings the pulp of his thumb into action so that the size, firmness, mobility, and temperature of this mass may be judged. The nature of that information will determine the next step in the operation. An assistant has chosen to use two double skin hooks to elevate the breast and retract the skin flap during this palpation process. This "feeling" process will tell the surgeon much about what is required for the next step in dissection.

When enlarging a pocket at some depth within the tissues, the surgeon may elect to dissect with the index fingers of both hands. In Figure 4.2 the surgeon is using this type of bimanual finger dissection. He fully pronates both forearms as he inserts his hands. With the dorsa of his hands braced against each other, he is able to use the powerful long flexor tendons of his forearms to exert maximum power at his fingertips to separate dense tissue. As he flexes both index fingers, their tips spread the tissues and enlarge the pocket in this breast with minimal trauma and bleeding. The fingers may then be advanced and the process repeated if an even deeper or larger pocket is needed.

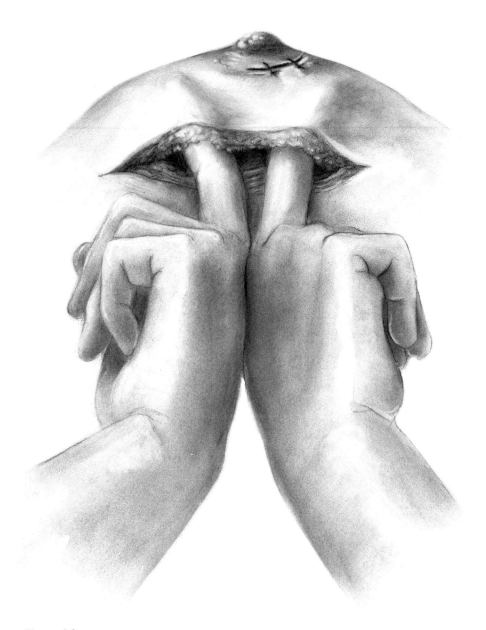

**Figure 4.2**

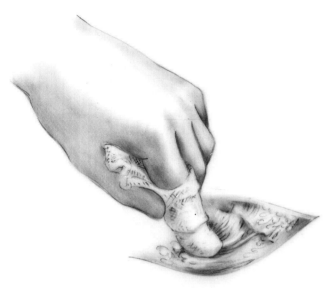

**Figure 4.3**

## Sponge or Gauze Dissection

Sometimes tissue density and adherence are sufficiently great that the moist gloved finger will not open the desired pocket. If a damp gauze sponge is wrapped about the surgeon's index finger as shown in Figure 4.3, the coefficient of friction between fingertip and wound will be increased. If the width of the wound permits, several extended fingers of the surgeon's hand may be jointly applied to the sponge so that a broad line of tissue dissection results from a single sweep of the hand. Figure 4.4 shows the surgeon using blunt gauze and four fingers to elevate and dissect the soft tissues of the face from the underlying periosteum of the mandible. The motion of dissection should be a firm push and rotation of the fingertips,

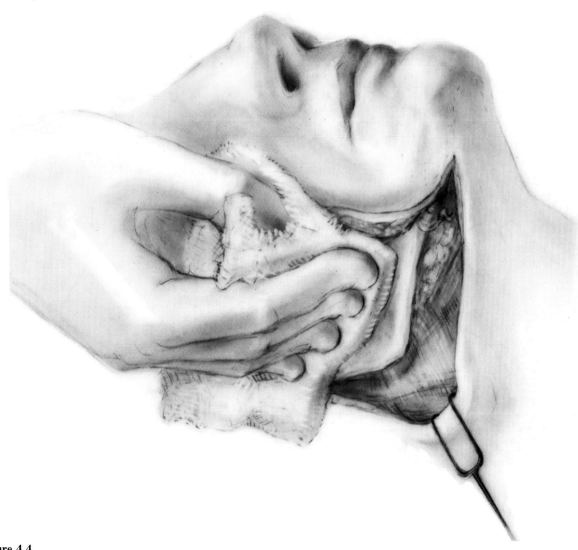

**Figure 4.4**

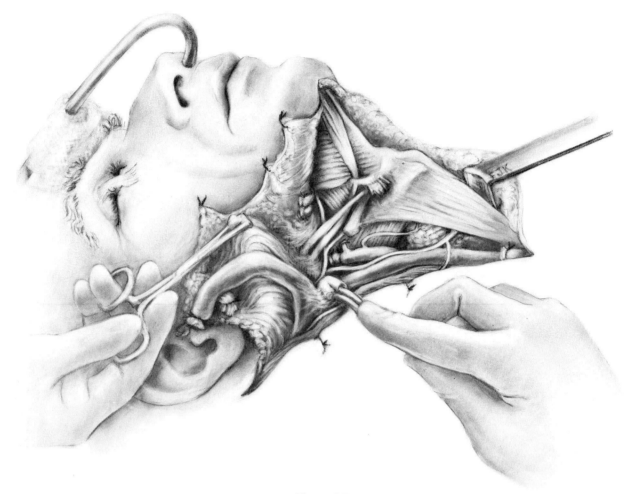

**Figure 4.5**

starting with the fingers on the deeper or more fixed tissue and followed by supinating the hand and wrist so as to lift and strip the more mobile tissue away from its deep attachments to the more fixed area at the leading angle of the dissection.

Gauze instrument dissection may be appropriate in narrow spaces where the surgeon may have difficulty inserting his hand. In such areas, a small rolled ''peanut'' of gauze (a Küttner pledget) is placed in the jaws of a Kocher clamp. The clamp, now tipped with this firm gauze nosepiece, is used to open the fascia in the same manner as when gauze is wrapped over an index fingertip. In Figure 4.5 the surgeon is doing a radical neck dissection, and using a gauze peanut to separate the internal jugular vein from the common carotid artery. The surgeon's index finger is extended along the clamp to a point near its tip. This increases his ability to apply force to the pledget as a firm supination of his wrist slides the pledget along the surface of the carotid wall to elevate the carotid sheath fascia and the jugular vein. The assistant lifts the sternomastoid muscle and node-bearing fascia (to be removed) laterally with the aid of a sharp-jawed clamp to help open the tissue plane.

This ''peanut'' dissection is more effective when the gauze pledget is folded in half before clamping (in the manner shown in Figure 4.6). The doubled pledget provides a larger, firmer, and more rounded dissecting surface to the tissues.

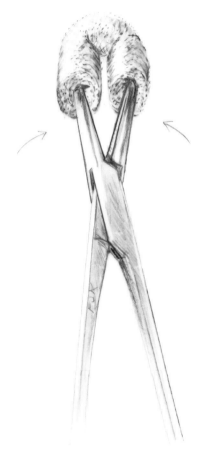

**Figure 4.6**

## Scissors Dissection

The use of the scissors for dissection is described in some detail in Chapter 2. In general, blunt-tipped scissors are excellent for opening tissue planes whenever those tissues are too dense for finger or sponge dissection, and not so dense as to require a scalpel. The wedging open of the tissues by repeated spreading of the blades of the scissors may be followed by dividing (under direct vision) of any tough residual fascial bands. This sequence of "spread, then look" makes this form of scissor dissection both safe and rapid in the hands of experienced surgeons. The shearing action of the scissor blades will close off and seal many small blood vessels at the moment they are cut. In many parts of the body this closure of the blades will result in less bleeding than when the same dissection is performed with a scalpel.

Dissection with sharp-tipped or double-edged scissors is indicated in special areas where tissue planes are parted with more difficulty.

## Knife Dissection

A sharp knife edge is needed for dissection whenever tissue is heavily scarred or very dense. Unlike the blunt-tipped scissors, a sharp knife will cut soft tissue with relative ease. It must therefore be directed with exact visual monitoring, or it may cause unexpected damage to normal important structures.

A dull knife is a very dangerous instrument! The heavy pressure required to make it divide tissue will make the cutting uncertain, and the surgeon will find it difficult to withdraw this pressure quickly enough, once the appropriate depth of cut has been reached. At times hospitals purchase "lowest bid" supplies of dull knife blades, or blades of a brand that become dull after only a few strokes. If a surgeon encounters such a blade, he should politely but firmly discard it and ask for another. He owes that much to his patient.

## Press Cutting

The stroking knife edge cannot be used as safely as the scissors tips as a method of palpating and finding a particular plane of dissection. However, if the edge of the scalpel is held stationary and gently pressed downward without stroking, it will nicely part any encountered collagen fibers that are under tension. Done carefully, this technique will spare underlying normal nerves and blood vessels and allow the surgeon to penetrate scar of unknown depth without damage to important underlying structures. In Figure 4.7 the scarred hand is being spread and held flat by the two hands of the assistant so that the cicatrix in the central palm is under marked tension. The fingers are extended and the palm widened by flattening the transverse metacarpal arch. The surgeon is holding the knife in a modified power grip to facilitate a simple downward pressure on the belly of the knife edge. No horizontal stroking motion of the blade is used. As the knife divides the stretched cicatrix, there is an almost audible "popping" of the strands. When the blade reaches underlying unscarred tissue, resistance to the knife blade stops, and the edge can be felt to gently displace the underlying normal tissues. After several of these parallel cicatricotomies are completed, the residual scar between the openings may be safely resected with scissors or knife to complete the release of the deep structures of the hand. Note that silk sutures have been used as retractors of the small flaps of palmar skin so as to free up the assistant's hands for other actions.

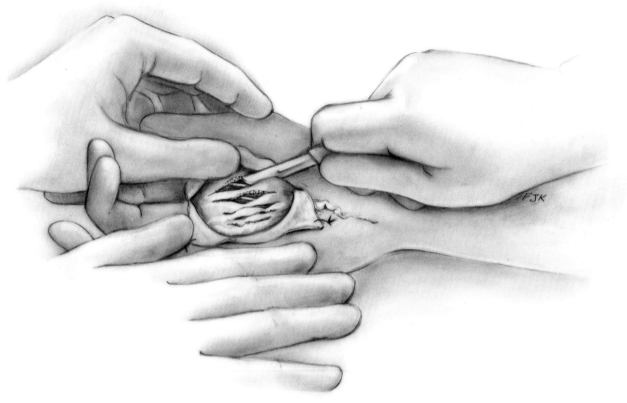

**Figure 4.7**

This author was first introduced to this method of "press cutting" of scar under tension by Sterling Bunnell at the Valley Forge General Hospital in 1945. Bunnell was fond of referring to scar tissue as "cancer of the hand" because of the way it infiltrated the delicate anatomy and immobilized the fine movements of the fingers. He advocated that the surgeon, whenever it was possible for him to do so, should dissect into scarred areas by approaching from normal tissue into areas where anatomy had been made abnormal by scar. Unfortunately, at times the badly damaged hand will not permit this "known-to-unknown" approach. In such cases, this method of press cutting with the knife allows us to find a safe way through dense scar without damaging the immediately subjacent digital nerves and vessels.

Most scalpel dissection is best performed with a smooth horizontal stroke that delivers even pressure along the entire cutting edge. Short strokes with uneven pressure on the knife blade cause additional tissue damage, increase bleeding, and increase operating time (see Chapter 1). They are usually a reflection of indecision on the part of the surgeon.

Some scalpel blades have double edges so that they will cut on any lateral movement of the blade. Others have a button or olive tip on the end of the blade so that cutting will only occur as a result of lateral sweeping of the blade. Three special-purpose scalpels are shown in Figure 4.8.

The olive-tip or "button-ended" knife (Fig. 4.8A) may be inserted in a narrow space and used to make only a lateral cut, while the rounded tip prevents any undesired damage from a blade point. Thus, the insertion of this knife into a pocket is safe and easy.

The Freer knife (Fig. 4.8B) has a rounded edge at its tip, and the cutting is limited to that precise area. It is of particular value in tangential undercutting to raise skin or mucous membrane. It combines some of the features of a knife edge with that of a sharp elevator.

The double-edged knife in Figure 4.8C has both a sharp tip and a sharp edge on both sides. It may be placed in a pocket and swept from side to side for rapid undermining. The sharp tip allows the surgeon to advance this blade into relatively dense tissue (unlike the button-ended knife). These and other special knife blades are only needed for unusual circumstances.

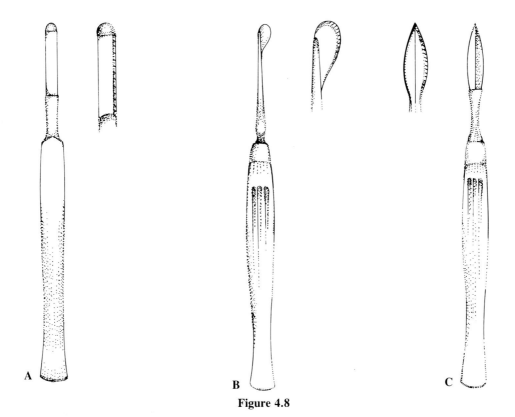

**Figure 4.8**

## Laser Dissection

Surgical lasers are beams of light of coherent wavelength. They carry intense and concentrated energy. When the correct wavelength is chosen (argon), the laser (argon) energy is absorbed by red cells in vessels of the skin. Other wavelengths (the $CO_2$ laser) will cause the skin to vaporize along the line of incision. Small (but not large) diameter blood vessels are also coagulated by the heat as the skin is divided. Lasers have been used since the early 1970s for surgical dissection. These intense, tiny, powerful beams of coherent light, like sharp scalpels, have the capacity to divide tissue with minimal damage to the cells on either side of the incision. Since these beams may be reflected by mirrors, this cutting capacity may be reflected around corners or into cavities (i.e., laryngeal lesions) that are hard to reach with a scalpel.

The surgical laser may in the future become an important surgical tool for dissection, but at present there are several drawbacks. The process is still quite slow compared to a scalpel, the equipment is expensive and space-consuming, eye protection must be provided to all in the operating room, and repair service for the laser is not always readily available. Until physiological advantages such as improved hemostasis or better wound healing can be demonstrated, it is unlikely that laser dissection will become

the norm. However, even now, the removal of certain highly vascular lesions such as lymphangiomas may be accomplished with reduced blood loss by use of the laser.

## Electrocautery Dissection

Unlike the laser, the electrosurgical unit has stood "the test of time." It is a valuable and established method of hemostasis in most surgical specialties (see Chapter 5).

The electrosurgical unit is used by some surgeons both for surgical dissection and for hemostasis. When large incisions are made, or large flaps of skin or muscle are elevated, the cutting cautery may be of significant value.

In dissecting with the cutting current, the frequency of current should be adjusted so that minimal tissue coagulation occurs. When a bleeding vessel is severed, the surgeon may momentarily switch to coagulation to obtain hemostasis. The cutting current will not differentiate between dense and loose tissue planes. It will cut whatever soft tissue it touches. It does not allow the surgeon any sense of palpation in seeking his plane. Like the scalpel, it must be carefully controlled by visual monitoring. It is, consequently, less useful in dissections through areas of distorted anatomy. Both experimental and clinical observations would indicate that postoperative wound seromas are more common after dissection by electrocautery than after knife or scissor dissection.

### The Hemostatic (Shaw) Scalpel

The hemostatic scalpel (Fig. 4.9) is a recent attempt to combine some of the advantages of a sharp knife and dissection with a heated blade. Many surgeons prefer not to use the hot blade to incise the skin, as the heat damages additional cells and makes the scar more noticeable. When set at 220°F, the blade can be used to part deeper tissues with reduced blood loss. The heat will seal small blood vessels as they are divided. The process is a slow form of dissection, and it is not yet clear that the method will be popular.

This instrument has proved of value in the carving and shaping of silastic and other alloplastic implants at the time of surgery. The heat in the blade facilitates carving these dense materials.

## Role of the Surgical Assistant

The chief surgeon will choose whichever blunt or sharp instrument he prefers at each stage of dissection. The good assistant will wish to facilitate the process of opening up of tissue planes to provide good exposure. In the preceding chapters we have indicated many actions that the assistant surgeon may take to help the surgeon when scalpel, scissors, or retractors are being used.

As dissection proceeds to deeper tissues, the surgical spotlights usually need to be redirected at different angles to better illuminate the wound. The treasured assistant will quietly attend to this without waiting for a request from the surgeon. If only a single light is on the working field, he must always take care to avoid moving it completely off the field and plunging the work area into darkness in the process of adjustment of the light. If temporary darkening of the field is required to improve the lighting, the surgeon should be warned in advance.

As the operation proceeds, constant, unobtrusive shifting or repositioning of the second assistant's retractors may be indicated. Any exposed tissues in inactive areas of the wound should be covered with moist packs or sponges to prevent cell damage from dessication. Cut suture ends and loose instruments should be removed from the field whenever a pause permits.

The first assistant should strive, with the least possible interruption, to manage hemostasis as the operation proceeds. This may involve having suction, clamps, scissors, ties, or the electrocautery poised and used at the proper moment.

Very often the surgical assistant can be quite helpful if he places countertraction on the tissues as the dissection continues. This stabilizes the point of instrument contact and usually frees up one of the operator's hands. Tamponading of any bleeding surface with simple pressure of finger, gauze, or pad should be almost a reflex motion by the surgical assistant.

In all operations, the assistant must remain alert and responsive. He should constantly be aware of all dangers to the patient and the needs of the precious living tissues for moisture and gentle handling. He should try hard to anticipate the very next step the surgeon will take and plan in advance of that step what action he may use to facilitate the process. If the surgical assistant makes, as it were, a game of always being ready, he will enjoy assisting and, in turn, will himself become a better chief surgeon.

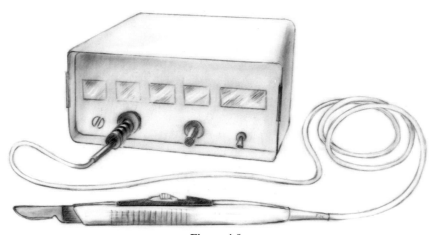

**Figure 4.9**

# 5

# Hemostasis and Removal of Blood From the Surgical Field

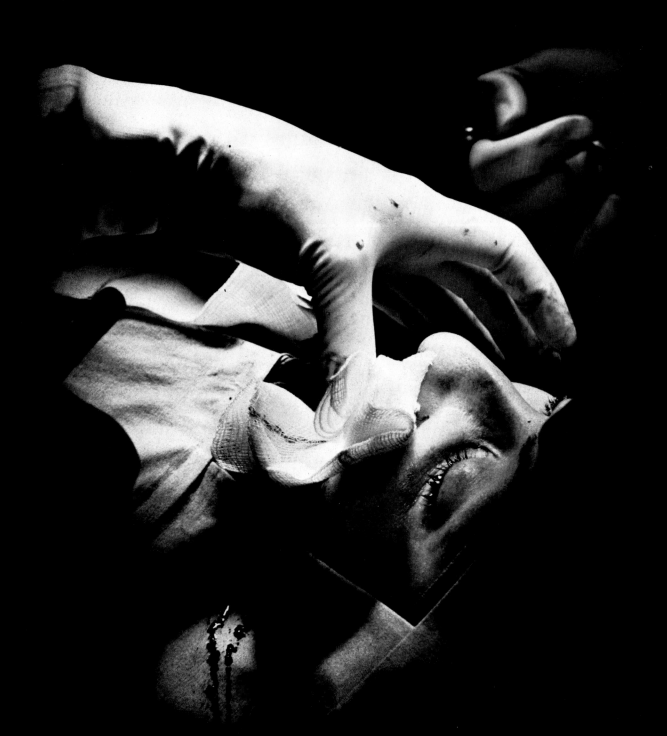

# 5

# Hemostasis and Removal of Blood From the Surgical Field

## Historical Methods of Arresting Bleeding

The modern surgeon seeks to prevent blood loss, in the first instance, by anticipatory control of vessels before they are divided. He then uses many methods to arrest as quickly as possible any bleeding that does occur. Once bleeding is stopped, he removes any residual liquid or clotted blood from the surgical wound before closure. Finally, he takes steps to minimize the chance of postoperative bleeding once the wound is closed. These composite actions to minimize blood loss during and after surgery constitute the art and science of hemostasis.

Excessive loss of blood may cause systemic complications such as shock, clotting disorders, anemia, or impaired wound healing. Leaving even small amounts of blood within a wound will reduce the visibility throughout the surgical field during the operation, provide a culture medium for bacteria, and, on breakdown of clots and red cells, chemically damage the adjacent tissues during the postoperative period.

In some surgical operations, hemostasis may be so difficult that it will require as much as 80% of the time and energies of the surgical team! There is thus a major premium on selection of the simplest and most appropriate techniques for obtaining good hemostasis.

Galen (130–200 A.D.) described several methods of controlling bleeding. He advocated both the use of direct pressure on bleeding points and, at times, the use of a hook to twist the end of a divided vessel and its adjacent tissues. He also described ligation of arteries with fiber. In some instances, he urged the application of styptics. All of these ancient techniques have a role in modern hemostasis. Unfortunately, Galen's sound teachings on this subject were ignored by many generations of doctors between his time and ours. Many of his principles had to be rediscovered. It is a reminder that even good surgical techniques may go unappreciated or be forgotten with changing trends in medicine!

## Modern Methods of Arresting Bleeding

### Hemostasis by Pressure

**Direct occlusion of hole in vessel by fingertip**

When an incision is made through skin, the surgeon or his assistant should instinctively and automatically place his fingertips or a moistened sponge against the opened ends of any transected and bleeding vessels. If this digital pressure is maintained for 15 to 20 seconds, small clots will usually form in the ends of many smaller vessels that have been divided, and no further bleeding will occur. The smooth surface of a gloved finger is less likely than the adherent surface of a gauze sponge to dislodge these fresh thrombi when the finger is removed. When gauze that has been applied to a bleeding point is withdrawn, the interlaced fresh clot may be pulled away with the sponge, and bleeding may begin anew (Fig. 5.1).

At the moment of removing any sponge or packs, the surgical team should be poised to control any renewed bleeding from larger divided vessels that had been occluded by the pressure.

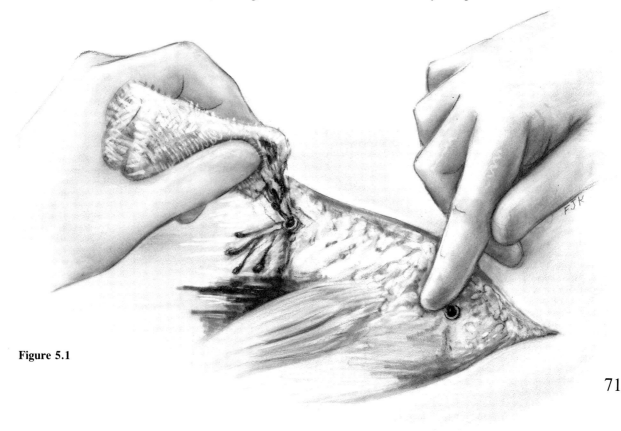

**Figure 5.1**

71

**Pressure against underlying bone**

When incised skin edge on one side of the wound happens to lie above bone, the surgeon's hand or a sponge may be placed on the external surface of that wound edge to compress the divided vessels against the firm underlying surface. Slight or partial serial release of that pressure will then allow identification, one by one, of the open ends of any larger vessels as spurts or drops of blood appear at the cut ends of each.

In Figure 5.2 the surgeon has placed the fingers of his left hand over the just-incised forehead skin. He quickly presses the skin down against the underlying bone to arrest any bleeding from the cut margin. He has released the index finger pressure just enough to allow a branch of the supraorbital artery to identify itself by bleeding. He is now about to grasp the end of this vessel with his fine-toothed Wainstock forceps (held in his right hand). As soon as the first assistant sees that the vessel end is secured by the forceps, he assures himself that no part of the metal forceps is touching any part of the wound except the vessel. Only then will he activate the audible buzz of the electrocautery and lightly touch any accessible metallic part of the forceps to coagulate the arterial opening. He should watch the vessel and forceps tips during coagulation to avoid continuation of the current beyond that needed to just seal the vessel. Excessive heat will cause more tissue necrosis and delay healing.

The surgeon will then reduce the pressure on his left long finger, and any bleeding vessels in that segment of the skin incision will be similarly spotted, grasped, and cauterized. This serial release of finger pressure is gentle, rapid, and efficient in minimizing blood loss.

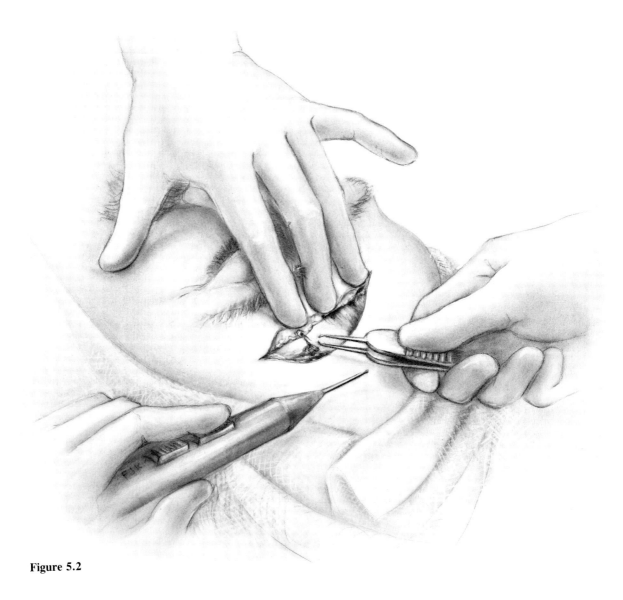

**Figure 5.2**

### Bidigital compression (pinch method)

When no underlying bone is present, but the soft tissues containing the bleeding vessels are mobile, the same technique of pressure occlusion and gradual release may be accomplished by squeezing the entire thickness of soft tissue (through which the trunk of a feeder artery passes) between the thumb and fingers of the nondominant hand. This method is seen in Figure 5.3 as the surgeon removes a cancer of the lip. In this illustration, he uses his nondominant left hand to compress the large right labial and nasolabial arteries. The first assistant is also using the thumb and index fingertips of his left hand to compress the patient's left labial artery. The lip tumor is then resected with a bloodless field. Once the specimen has been re-moved, a sequential release of finger-thumb pressures allows the precise location and control of all significant divided vessels. Note the manner in which the operator steadies his knife hand by resting his right little and ring fingers on the assistant's left index finger as the lip tissues are precisely divided. Small triphenylmethane dye dots (such as methylene blue) have been placed by puncture marks with a #25 hypodermic needle at the skin-vermilion junctions on either side of the excision. These dots will aid the surgeon in alignment of the lip in suture closure. The dye is slowly absorbed and the method is quite atraumatic to the tissues.

Whenever the surgeon realizes that a particular bleeding vessel is so large that it will require some

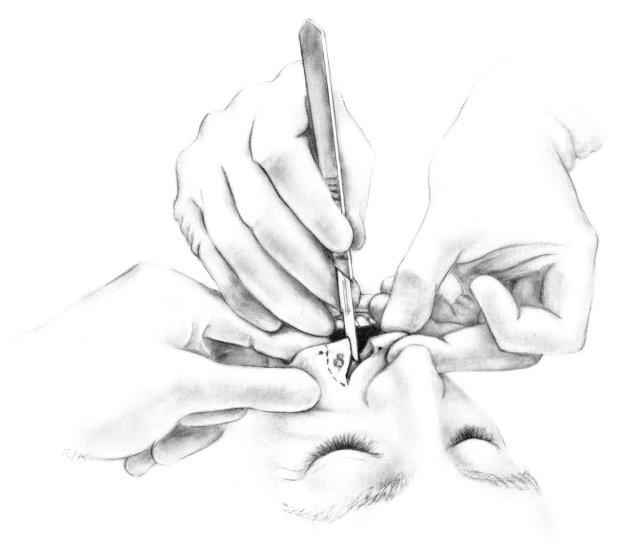

**Figure 5.3**

definitive hemostatic action later in the operation, it is usually best to obtain definitive hemostasis when the vessel is first divided. This early action will reduce total blood loss and allow some time for observation before final wound closure. That interval will verify the long-term effectiveness of the hemostatic method used and reduce the risk of postoperative bleeding.

### Pressure with knife or instrument tip

Often the surgeon may simply use the tip of his knife to immediately compress the open lumen of an artery that reveals its presence by spurting just as the knife has transected it. In Figure 5.4 the knife pauses and the tip of the blade is quickly redirected to cover the cut vessel and stop the blood loss until the assistant can arrive with clamp or forceps and is prepared to grasp and cauterize the bleeding point when the knife blade is removed. The tip of a suction cannula may also be used in a similar manner by the surgical assistant to momentarily compress and arrest a bleeding point.

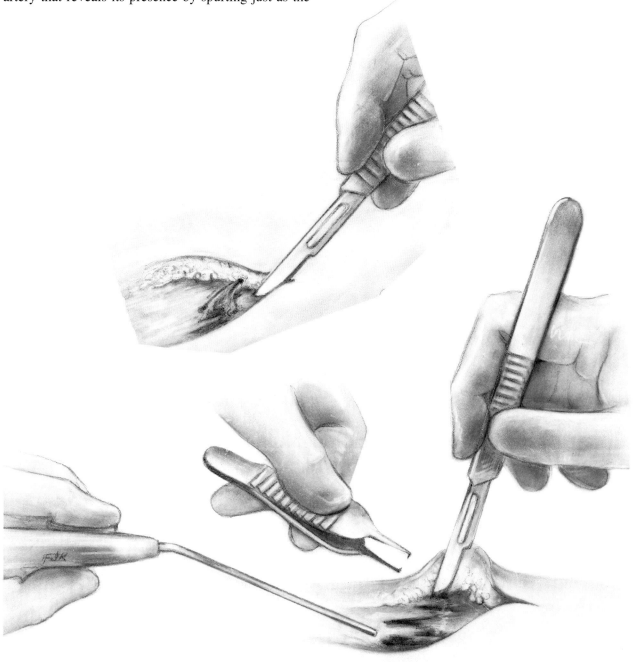

**Figure 5.4**

## Sponge and sponge stick pressure

Sponges may be applied directly to bleeding surfaces by the hand and fingers in order to arrest bleeding. At times, however, a bleeding point arises in a deep hole or recess, and the operator needs a long-handled instrument to reach the vessel and apply pressure with the sponge until he is ready to clamp, ligate, or cauterize.

In Figure 5.5 the surgeon is using a sponge stick—a small gauze pack fixed in a long-handled clamp with looped, teardrop-shaped jaws—to place pressure against a bleeding point in a deep recess behind the cecum and the ascending colon. The sponge stick is held in position until retractors and lighting are in good position. Any loose blood is then cleared away by suction, while the surgeon or assistant obtains a long artery clamp to secure the cut end of the vessel. Only then is the sponge stick rolled slowly off the vessel to expose its cut end for clamping.

## Pressure by packing

In some operations, diffuse bleeding may require pressure for an extended period for good control. In such circumstances, a moist pack may be pressed against the bleeding surface for 10 to 20 minutes while some other part of the operation is completed. The saline used to moisten the pack should be cool, not warm. Contrary to earlier popular beliefs, firm experimental data show that warm compresses *on bleeding surfaces will increase the amount of blood loss*. The widespread idea that warm saline might reduce bleeding by increasing the rate of clotting has proved to be erroneous.

Dry packs stop bleeding well, but they cause tissue dessication and tend to adhere to the newly formed clots. These fresh clots may be pulled free on removal of the pack and reopen bleeders. Dry gauze is also more injurious than moist gauze when applied to the cells and tissues of any wound. In rare in-

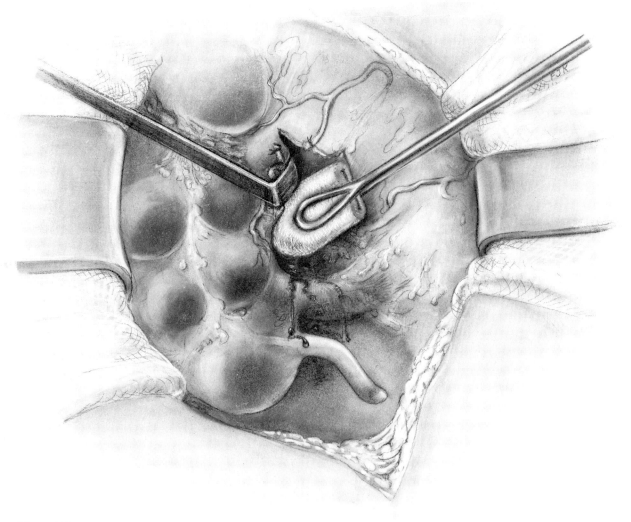

**Figure 5.5**

stances, a wound pack must be left in place for 10 days as the only practical method of arresting a particularly aggressive hemorrhage. This long-term packing of the wound is most likely to be required in the partial removal of a large arteriovenous malformation.

If troublesome bleeding arises from a deep recess where the open end of the vessel may not be seen, a small sponge clamped in a ring clamp (sponge stick), as shown in Figure 5.5, may be used to reach "around the corner" and tamponade the bleeding vessel in the hidden area. Here the sponge stick compresses a branch of the right colic artery while the wound is enlarged to expose and clamp the offending vessel. It is a mistake to try to get control of deep bleeding without first obtaining adequate exposure.

## Hemostasis by Twist Occlusion

In some tissues, the elastic density of fascia about a divided artery of medium size makes it practical to control bleeding by twist occlusion. The surgeon simply clamps the divided end of the artery along with some of the adjacent fascia with a straight or curved artery clamp. He then slowly rotates the shaft of the clamp for five or six complete turns with the tip of his index finger as illustrated in Figure 5.6A. After several turns the clamp tip may spontaneously separate from the tissues. The twisting action will usually cause closure and retraction of the artery and succeed in stopping the bleeding. The rotary twirling motion of the hand, with the index finger inserted through one ring of the artery clamp as shown in Figure 5.6B, is a rapid and efficient technique for twisting. This so-called "French twist" method has the advantage of leaving no ligated or coagulated tissue that requires later cleanup by the wound phagocytes. It should not be used as the sole means of hemostasis on arteries with diameters of more than 1 to 2 mm.

## Hemostasis by Ligatures and Metal Clips

### Types of ligatures

Large, discrete blood vessels may not stop bleeding even after pressure, packs, or twisting. In Greece, during the period of Alexander (first and second centuries B.C.), physicians had already learned to control bleeding from cut blood vessels by tying them with ligatures made from strands of natural biologic materials such as fiber and cloth. In today's surgery, a great variety of synthetic alloplastic materials are also used to tie off blood vessels. Ligatures and sutures are today the mainstays for obtaining hemostasis of

large vessels, just as electrocoagulation has become the method of choice with control of bleeding from smaller vessels.

The ligation of divided arteries and veins may be achieved by the use of either absorbable or nonabsorbable materials. Nonabsorbable materials are defined as those that will remain in the tissues for 60 days or longer. They may be flexible (silk, cotton, nylon, etc.) or rigid (metal clips). Nonabsorbable ligatures may be prepared from natural materials or they may be synthesized.

Whatever material is used, the ligature should be applied about the circumference of the bleeding vessel and its adventitia as closely as possible to its divided end. When larger bites of tissue are included within the tie, a larger and stronger material is needed, the resulting knot is bulkier, and additional living tissue will be strangulated and forced to undergo subsequent necrosis. *Gross technique leads to gross results.* A brawny, lumpy, red wound after surgery is often a reflection of rough technique, heavy-handed use of the cautery, grasping large bites of tissue in clamps, applying sutures too tightly, and poor approximation of tissue. Patients deserve better.

Good surgeons may choose to use either absorbable or nonabsorbable ties. Both have advantages and disadvantages. In general, the reduced break strength (for a corresponding diameter) and greater tissue reactivity of catgut (natural collagen) and dexon (synthetic collagen) have led me to prefer a stronger nonabsorbable material of smaller diameter such as silk or nylon in ligating vessels. Absorbable suture materials also lack some of the flexibility and handling qualities of silk and other nonabsorbable materials.

Although silk continues to have the best "hand qualities" and knot-setting accuracy of all surgical sutures, its multistrandedness and associated large total surface area cause the wound to produce more fibrosis about it than about a monofilament nylon suture of comparable strength. For many years, I have found that 5-0, 4-0, and 3-0 clear nylon is excellent for buried sutures or ties. Nylon produces little tissue reaction. The setting of the knot requires slightly more precision and care with nylon than with silk. Since silk cuticular sutures are usually removed after 5 to 7 days its tissue reactivity is just becoming evident at that time and, with such early removal, causes little disadvantage to the healing wound.

### An all-purpose two-handed tie

There are several commonly used methods of placing one-handed and two-handed ties about the end

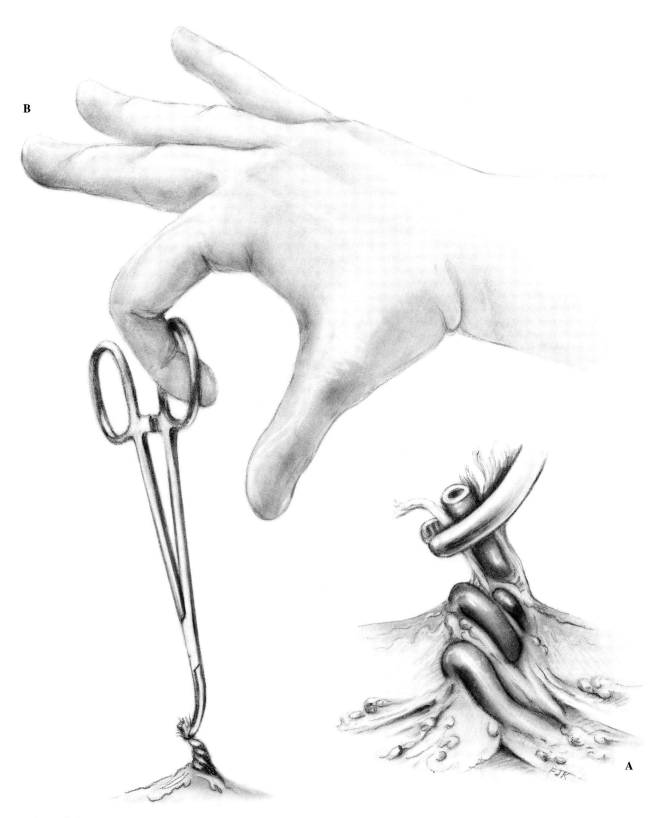

**Figure 5.6**

of a clamped vessel. The young surgeon should give some thought to desirable criteria for the method of tying that he will choose to adopt.

Any ideal method of tying knots should allow continuous control of both ends of the ligature. The ideal method also would not require visual location of a loose suture end (this is of special importance when using very fine or noncolored suture materials). It is also important that a method of tying be chosen in which the hands of the surgeon do not obstruct the assistant surgeon's view of the tip of the instrument that is clamped on the vessel that is being ligated. A clear view of the clamp tip is needed, especially at the moment when the first throw of the knot is laid flat and tightened. An unobstructed view at that instant allows the assistant to properly time his gradual release of the clamp just as the surgeon increases tension on the first knot. As the clamp is slowly opened, the ligature gathers up the clamped vessel and fascia into a circular cross-section.

Only one technique of knot tying meets all of these requirements. Most surgeons in early training watch their seniors tie bleeders by reaching an empty hand behind an elevated clamp that is holding a vessel. They then use the fingers of that hand to grasp the free end of a tie that is passed to it by the other hand (Fig. 5.7). With this method of beginning his tie, the surgeon finds that, regardless of his next movements, he must cross his hands in order to lay his first throw flat as the first knot is tied. This crossing of his hands occurs at the exact moment that will impair his clamp-holding assistant's view of the knot—that is, just at the time of clamp release. This often results in an inaccurate and poorly timed release—either too soon or too late.

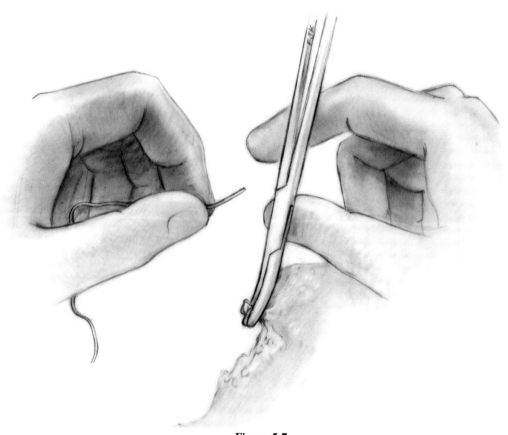

**Figure 5.7**

The First Throw

All of this may be avoided if, from the beginning, the surgeon develops the habit of carrying the short end of his tie behind the clamp with his initial hand motion. This same motion should also guide the tie down low and close to the clamped vessel and clamp tip (Fig. 5.8A–B). The hand holding the short end of the tie should pass that end behind the nose of the clamp and, in the same motion, give it to the thumb and index fingers of the opposite (left) hand.

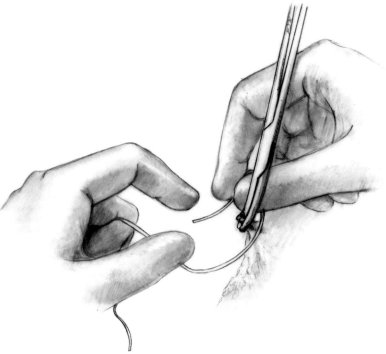

**Figure 5.8A**

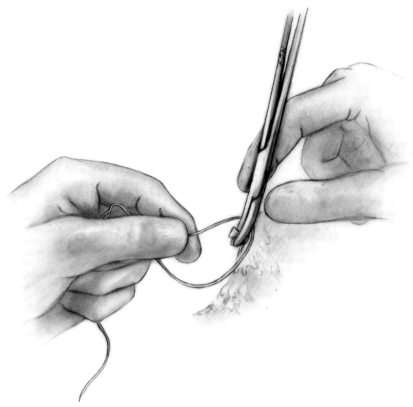

**Figure 5.8B**

If the tie is not also led down to the angle between the tissue and the clamp tip, but is instead passed about the clamp at mid-shaft level, the assistant may inadvertently pull the tie out of the operator's hands when he attempts to point up the nose of the clamp prior to tying the first knot. At the beginning of the tying, the surgeon has continued to grasp the long end of the ligature by the flexed long, ring, and little fingers of his left hand. This has left his left thumb-and-index pinch mechanism free to receive the short end of the ligature as it is passed behind the clamp with his right hand.

The right hand now regains the short end of the tie (Fig. 5.8B). The right hand releases the short end, moves to the front of the clamp and regains the short end from the left thumb and index fingers. The long and short ends are now encircling the clamped vessel and are already crossed as they are held in the operator's two hands (Fig. 5.8C).

The long finger of the right hand then pulls open a large loop by hooking its distal phalanx into the loop to the right. This makes it easy for the left index finger to curl downward through the opened loop and pinch the short end of the tie against the left thumb pulp (Fig. 5.8D).

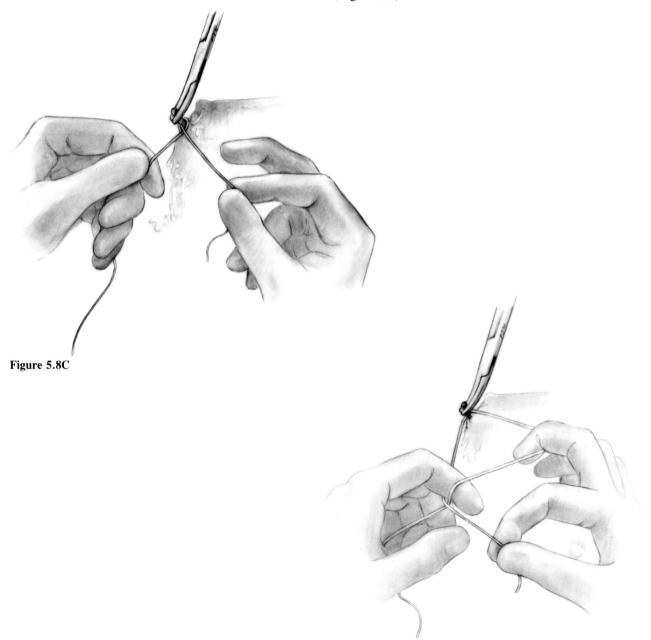

**Figure 5.8C**

**Figure 5.8D**

The left wrist is then pronated to deliver the left thumb and index and the short end of the tie upward through the still widely opened loop. The short end is now in good position to be grasped by pinching it between the thumb and index finger of the right hand as that hand is brought into the desired position by modest supination of the right wrist (Fig. 5.8E). The long finger of the right hand then releases the loop as the first knot is drawn tight. Note (Fig. 5.8F) that the surgeon's hands are not crossed as the first throw is tightened, and the assistant has an unobstructed view of the knot. This allows him to release the clamp just as the loop gathers up the tissue and the vessel held in the first throw of the ligature. The surgeon must avoid jerking or putting tension on either end of the tie from the time of setting the first knot until after he tightens the second. Tension on either end will loosen the first knot and let the bleeder pull free.

Once the two ends of the tie have been crossed and the first throw of the square knot has been pulled tight and flat, the second part of a standard loop-opening two-handed method completes a square knot.

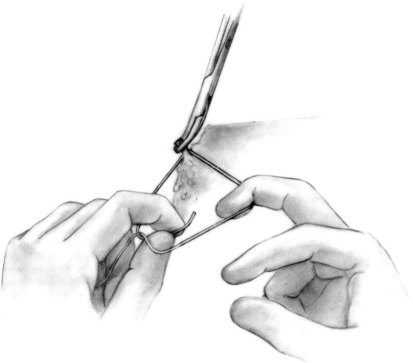

**Figure 5.8E**

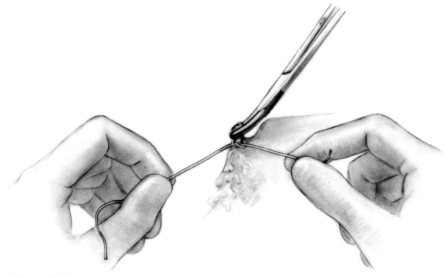

**Figure 5.8F**

The Second Throw

In Figure 5.9A the surgeon, having set the first throw of his knot, reaches above the short end of the tie (still held in the pinch between the thumb and index fingers of his right hand) and uses his right long and ring fingers to make a generous loop out of the long end of the tie. He then brings the short end around and up over the long end of the tie and into this loop with his right thumb and index fingers. It is held there until pinched between the pulps of his left thumb and index finger (Fig. 5.9B). The left thumb and index, now having control of the short end, bring it down through the loop by a flexing motion of the left wrist (Fig. 5.9C). The right thumb and index then again grasp the end, and the surgeon's hands are now in position to tighten the second throw.

To flatten this second knot for proper squaring, the surgeon must now cross his right hand over the knot as he tightens (Fig. 5.9D). In this instance, the crossover of the hand causes no "visual block" problem as the assistant has already released the clamp with the first throw.

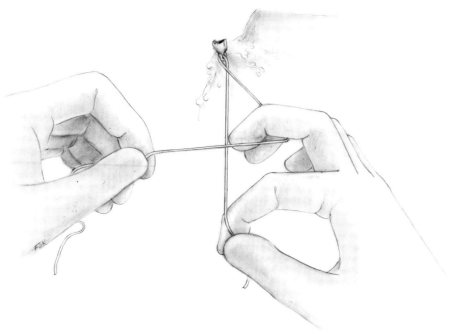

**Figure 5.9A**

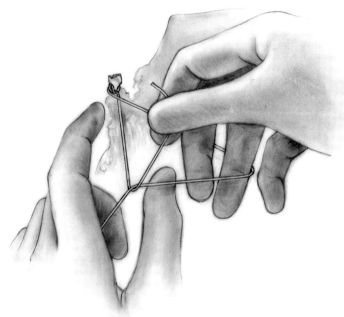

**Figure 5.9B**

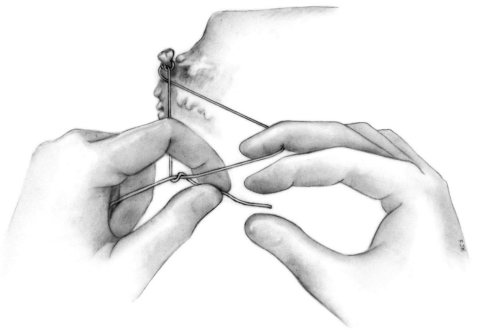

**Figure 5.9C**

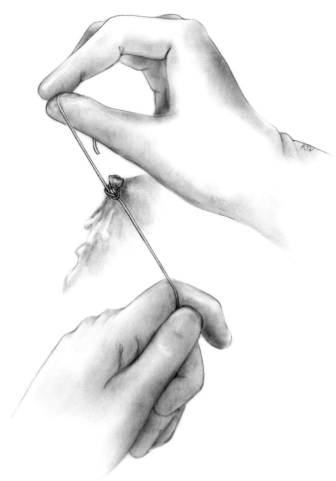

**Figure 5.9D**

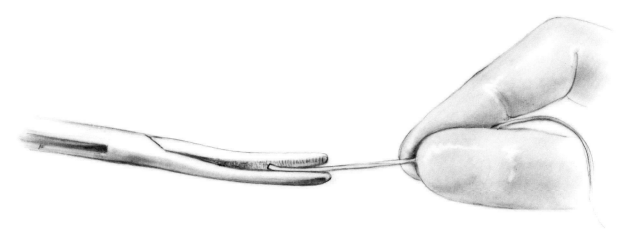

**Figure 5.10**

### Tie-on-a-clamp technique

While working on hemostasis of large vessels well below the skin surface, the surgeon will often request a "tie-on-a-clamp" from his scrub nurse. The end of the silk (or other material) tie should be clamped end-on by the nurse (Fig. 5.10) so that the tie emerges from the exact tip of a slightly curved clamp. Figure 5.11 shows a tie-on-a-clamp being passed behind a long-handled right-angled clamp that is controlling a bleeder in a deep hole. Note again, that the tie has been placed in the very tip of the jaws of the Kelly clamp so as to facilitate passage.

As the tie is pressed down behind the curved jaws of the right-angled clamp toward its tip at the level of the vessel, the surgical assistant, without releasing the vessel, tilts the right-angled clamp so that its tips point toward the operator. He also gently lifts them slightly above the level of the clamped vessel and adjacent tissue. Holding the clamp in that elevated position (Fig. 5.11) facilitates easy passage of the ligature and holds the first throw of the knot beneath the tips of the right-angled clamp. The surgeon may then choose to lengthen the short-end by drawing up sufficient suture to complete the knot with his fingers. If, however, the clamped vessel is in a deep and narrow recess he may choose, after placing the short end of the suture beneath the tip of the clamp to release the suture end from the passing clamp and use it to do an instrument tie (Fig. 5.12). The right-angled clamp is slowly released as the first knot is tightened by using the Kelly clamps to pull the short end of the ligature into the depths of the recess (Fig. 5.13).

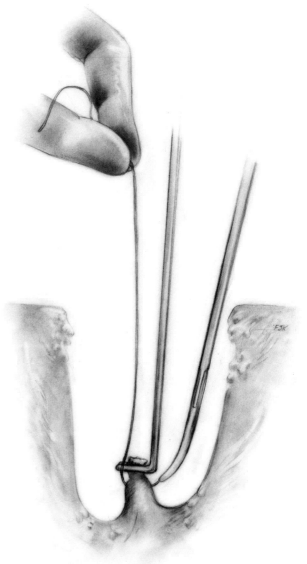

**Figure 5.11**

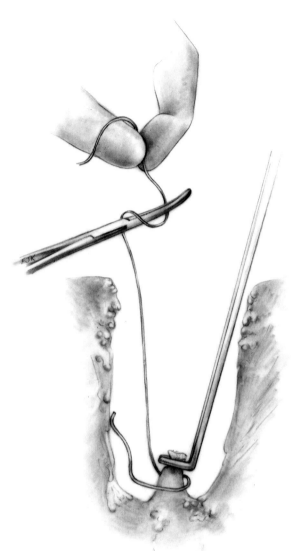

**Figure 5.12**

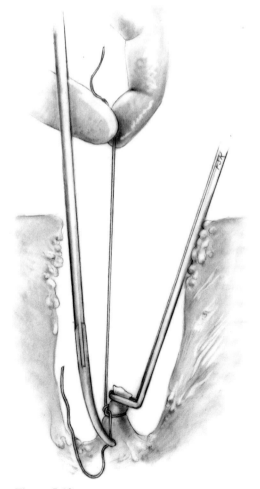

**Figure 5.13**

At times the clamp holding a bleeder happens to be positioned with its point facing a full 180° away from the surgeon. In such circumstances, especially if the clamped tissue has a broad base, it may be wise to leave the clamp facing at that angle while the first throw is tied as the assistant surgeon simply lifts upward the clamped vessels. The surgeon may then start the tie by using the tie-on-a-clamp to hook the silk beneath the nose of the right-angled clamp and then tie on the shaft side of that clamp. At this point, the surgeon is in position to execute an instrument tie to complete his knot (Fig. 5.14).

### Instrument tie-in-a-hole

When a vessel has been clamped in a deep recess or narrow hole, it may be possible for the surgeon to tie his knots by running his index finger down in the recess. At times his finger will not be long enough to reach the bottom of a narrow space and an instrument tie may be needed to place a firm ligature on the vessel stump. The principles are the same as for manual tie, except that the slender tip of a needle holder or a long-handled curved clamp (such as a Kelly) is substituted for one of the hands and the index finger of the operator. The Kelly clamp first passes the end of the tie about the tip of the clamp on the vessel. The short end is brought up so that its end is readily in view

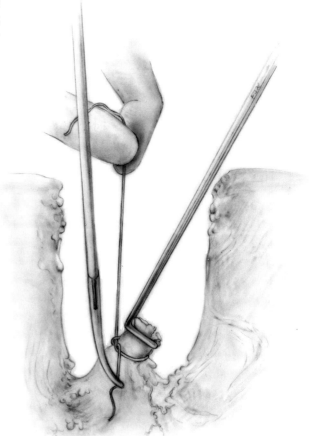

**Figure 5.14**

and then released. The Kelly is then brought to the surface of the wound and a loop in the long end of the suture is thrown about its tip (Fig. 5.15A). The tip of the Kelly is then directed downward (Fig. 5.15B)

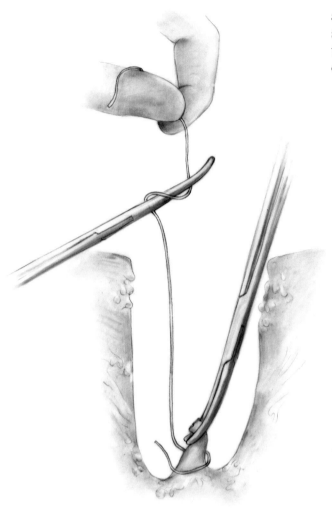

**Figure 5.15A**

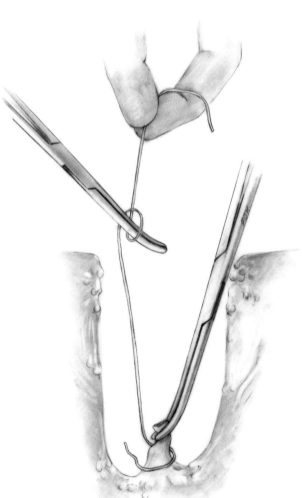

**Figure 5.15B**

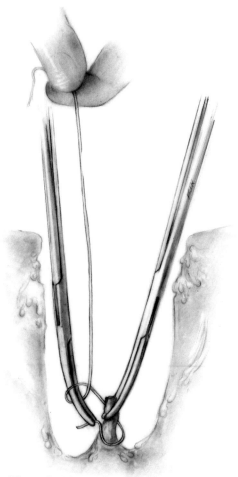

**Figure 5.15C**

and used to once again secure the short end on the depths of the wound (Fig. 5.15*C*). Once the short end is grasped by the clamp (Fig. 5.15*C*), it is used to tighten each throw by pushing the tip past the point of ligation to an even deeper part of the recess (Fig. 5.15*D*). If the short end is not in this manner pushed away from the wound surface when tightening the knot, the ligature is likely to be pulled off the tissue by an upward vector of force that is created when a pull is placed on *both* the short and long ends of the tie from points near the surface level of the wound.

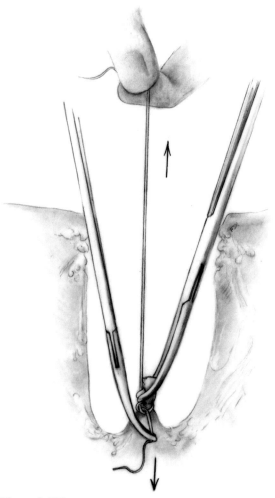

**Figure 5.15D**

As the first throw is tightened the tissue is released with removal of the clamp by the assistant. The surgeon once more returns the short end of the tie to a visible location (in a more superficial part of the wound) before releasing it (Fig. 5.16). He then throws a second loop into the long end of the tie as shown in Figure 5.17. He snugs down this second throw (Fig.

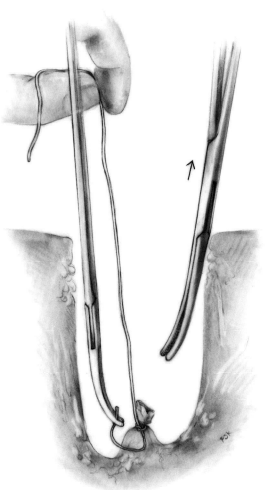

**Figure 5.16**

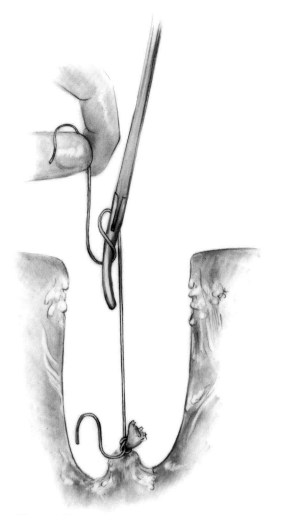

**Figure 5.17**

5.18) by placing a clamp on the long end of the ligature and pushing it downward so as to square the second knot. A second clamp is used to counter-pull the
short end of the tie toward the operator in a direction
180° away from the long end. Three or four throws
may be required.

As the inset in Figure 5.18 shows, the surgeon
must not tighten the second throw of his knot by
clamping and pushing the *short* end of his tie to the
base of the wound. To do so will cause him to fail to
lay a flat square knot.

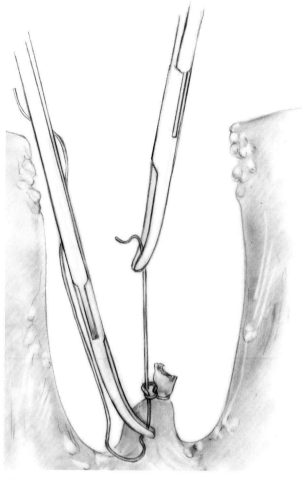

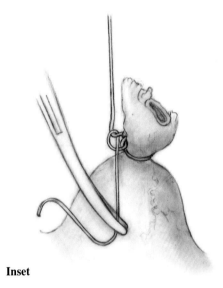

**Inset**                                    **Figure 5.18**

### Metallic clips

Metal clips are used by neurosurgeons and others
to control bleeding, seal dural leaks, or serve as mark-
ers in the postoperative period. The long handle of
the special clip holder allows the surgeon to reach
deep bleeders in narrow quarters. Tying ligatures may
be difficult in such spaces, and at times the use of the
electrocautery should be avoided as it may damage
adjacent neural tissue or fail to seal a larger vessel.

Metal clips can be applied rapidly, but it must
be possible to first lift and oppose the walls of the
vessel that is to be clipped (usually with the aid of a
second pair of forceps). Figure 5.19 shows a method
of clipping a large branch of a vessel. One clip has
been placed, and a second is about to be applied as
the lumen is pressed flat by a pair of forceps. The
vessel may then be divided between the two clips.

The stiff metal clips have a tendency to become
dislodged if used on highly mobile or pulsatile tissues.

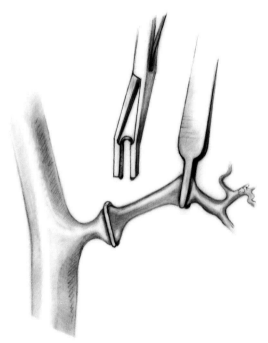

**Figure 5.19**

They are also radiopaque. This feature may be an advantage (as a marker) or a disadvantage as they interfere with the use of computed tomographic or magnetic resonance images in the postoperative period.

## Hemostasis by Suture Ligatures

### Placing of sutures through vessels

Larger veins and arteries often require transfixation with suture ligatures for secure control. Simple ties on the stumps of major arteries may be slowly dislodged by the continued pulsing of the column of blood against the tie. Both a tie and a suture ligature may be used on arteries to prevent this danger of postoperative bleeding. The suture should be placed more proximally, as its transfixation of the vessel wall will resist this displacement action of the pumping artery.

When the cut end of a vessel is clamped, it is helpful if the jaws of the clamp are allowed to extend 2 to 3 mm beyond the clamped tissue. This modest free projection of the tips of the clamp may be used to guide a silk tie or suture into position as it is passed. The projecting tips help retain the silk behind the clamp during tying. In Figures 5.11–5.17 the value of this method of clamping may be seen. In Figure 5.20A the needle has been passed through the midpart of the stalk of the clamped artery. In Figure 5.20B it completely encircles the clamped vessel before it is tied. As the tie is tightened (Fig. 5.20C), the first assistant will perform a gradual "educated" release of the clamp. This release allows the suture to gather up the clamped tissue and change its cross-section from a flattened to a circular form. In addition to the proper timing of his release, another action may be required of the assistant. If the position of the clamp has twisted the tissue, this twist should be slowly unrolled (the "educated" release) by the assistant just as the clamp jaws open. A too rapid release of the clamp will cause some vessels to escape the grip of the ligature.

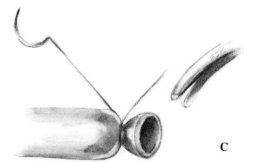

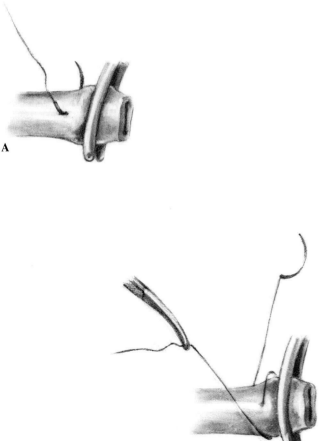

A

B

C

**Figure 5.20**

The all-purpose two-handed tie described and shown in Figures 5.8 and 5.9 gives excellent and secure control of knotting with both suture ligatures and ties. Once proficient in its use, the surgeon will find that it is as rapid a method of tying as any one-handed technique.

### Suture of buried bleeders

Some bleeding vessels, on sectioning, retract deeply into tissue and cannot be readily clamped. In such instances, a figure-eight or running lashing suture may be placed so as to produce localized constriction of the cut surface along with the vessel. In Figure 5.21 the surgeon has placed a figure-eight suture to encircle 8 or 10 venous sinusoids that are difficult to cauterize or ligate. If the suture is tied with proper tension, the bleeding will stop without producing strangulation and ischemic necrosis of the tissue included within the loops. At times a pledget of gel foam or another absorbable hemostatic material may be included in the loops of the suture to offer further tamponade. In Figure 5.22 the surgeon has used a large noncutting needle to place a criss-cross continuous suture across the margins of a bleeding surface of the liver after biopsy of a large vascular nodule. The suture is then tied down over a block of gel foam to compress and seal the vessels. The lobe of the liver has then been retracted for further surgery on the biliary tract.

### Temporary suture tourniquet of vessels in continuity

Sutures may also be used to control bleeding by temporarily placing them as tourniquets around vessels that are left in continuity. In Figure 5.23 the surgeon is about to operate on the left upper lip. He knows that the left external maxillary artery supplies the major circulation to that area. By placing a silk suture through the tissues near the oral commissure so as to encompass the feeder artery, he has been able to tie a slip knot that blocks much of the arterial flow to the lip. A clamp has been fixed to the loop and to the two free ends of the suture. It will be used during surgery as a lip retractor. Once the operation is completed, the slip knot is untied, the suture is removed, and the circulation is restored.

This technique of temporary suture occlusion of regional axial arteries is of much value about the head and neck where blood flow is so vigorous.

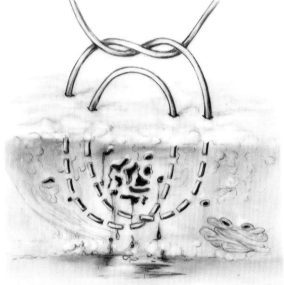

**Figure 5.21**

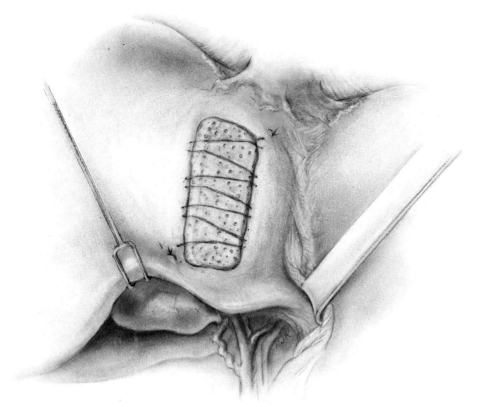

**Figure 5.22**

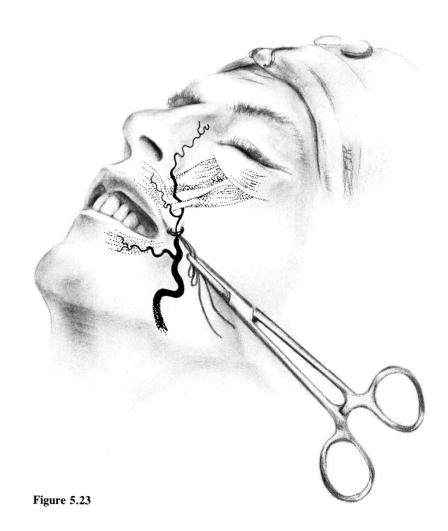

**Figure 5.23**

**Direct suture of vessel walls**

Very large or nonexpendable bleeding vessels such as the vena cava or the internal carotid artery are best controlled by direct repair of any breaks or rents in their walls. This may require simple suture (with a taper-pointed vascular needle) of the vessel wall, or a vascular clamp may be used to partially occlude the flow while a running suture is used to close the tear in the wall. Figure 5.24 shows simple repair of the wall of the internal carotid artery with a running non-absorbable suture. In suturing, the bites must be placed closely together to avoid leaking of blood when the Potts occlusion clamp (with multiple fine teeth to avoid crushing the vessel wall) is removed. Since the clamp has only partially occluded the vessel, blood flow to the brain has been maintained during the period of vessel repair.

**Patch repair of vessel walls**

A portion of the wall of a nonexpendable vessel may be lost as a result of trauma or following its resection to remove a cancer. It may be necessary to close the defect in the vessel wall with a patch graft from an autogenous expendable vein or artery to prevent undue narrowing of the lumen. In Figure 5.25 a patch of the internal jugular vein has been used to repair a defect in the common carotid artery after a radical neck dissection. The temporary shunt was placed to avoid cerebral ischemia while the carotid was clamped off and the repair was in progress. Retrograde flow from the external carotid artery into the internal (while the common carotid is clamped) will also provide some additional protection of the brain in this situation. Internal shunts may be helped by using elastic perivascular loops that compress the vessel walls against the catheter.

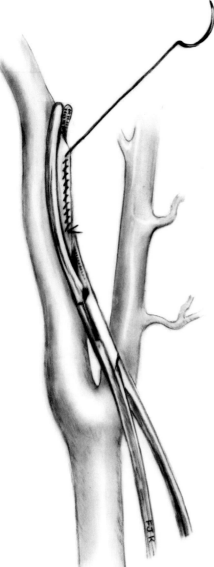

**Figure 5.24**

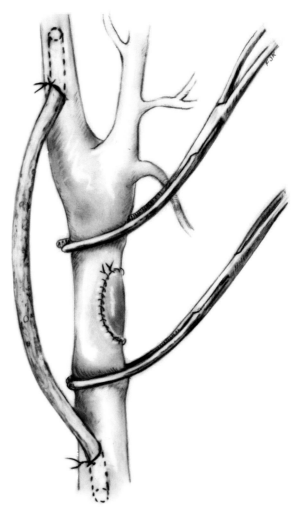

**Figure 5.25**

## Hemostasis by Cautery

### History

Even as recently as the early 1950s, many surgeons avoided extensive use of the electrocautery for wound hemostasis. The proper electrical frequency would coagulate protein and control bleeding by thrombosis of vessels, but damage to adjacent tissue was often noted to be quite extensive. On some occasions, the author has had the opportunity to reopen wounds 24 to 48 hours after the primary surgery. In some of these reopened wounds the size of the necrotic areas due to electrocoagulation of bleeders was astounding. Areas that had been cauterized lightly, leaving visible evidence of damage that seemed small and localized at the time of closure, showed, two days later, many sites of necrosis that were 5 to 8 mm in diameter! A surgeon cannot depend on visual evidence to determine accurately the amount of damage he inflicts with this risky tool.

In the 1940s, I had the pleasure of working closely with the late Grant Ward, a pioneer in the use of electrosurgery to treat cancer. He and Howard Kelly had written one of the classic textbooks on electrosurgery. In subsequent operations on large numbers of cancer paients, we used electrocautery to obtain hemostasis. When some of these cauterized wounds were immediately covered by skin grafts, serum and fluid accumulations frequently formed beneath the grafts in the immediate postoperative period. This degree of fluid formation was not seen when use of the cautery was deliberately avoided in patients with similar wounds who also received skin grafts.

With the passage of time, technical improvements in electrophysics have reduced some of the undesirable side effects of the Bovie units, but unrecognized tissue injury still occurs, and surgeons must school themselves and their assistants to take special precautions as they use this dangerous instrument. In many operations, its appropriate use will save much valuable operating time. The precise tip of the divided vessel is all that need be coagulated.

The bipolar cautery has been of special value to control small bleeders in delicate areas such as the eyelids and in all types of microvascular and microneural surgery.

The bipolar cautery also offers the advantage of permitting coagulation in a wet environment. The damage is also confined to the tissue between the tips of the cauterizing forceps. Its effectiveness is somewhat limited and slow when used to control large bleeders in extensive surgical wounds.

### Cautery techniques

When using the cautery for hemostasis, the power should be set at the lowest level commensurate with rapid localized vessel thrombosis. That level will depend on the size of the tissue bites clamped and offered by the surgeon or his assistant for coagulation. William Stewart Halsted taught surgeons to clamp the ends of individual vessels (with inclusion of minimal amounts of adjacent tissue) before tying them. We should strive for the same precision with electrocoagulation. A minimal amount of tissue should be lifted with the vessel. This means that very fine toothed forceps (Adson or Wainstock types) or mosquito clamps should be used.

The tissue about a vessel should be quite dry before cauterizing. The use of a fine suction tip to remove any blood, or a firm sponging just before applying the current, should be routine. An alert assistant will do this instinctively.

In Figure 5.26 the assistant would have been careful to have had the coagulation button ''on'' (with the sound monitor at proper level) *before* he touched the handle of the forceps. The delicate tips of this Adson-type forceps allow the precise limitation of the coagulation to the vessel and its immediate fascia. For very fine work, the Wainstock forceps (Fig. 3.8) provide even thinner teeth.

If the assistant touches the forceps with the cautery tip *before* turning on the current, he will find that it is much more difficult to judge and control the amount of current (time of application) with sufficient accuracy. If, however, the current is on at the moment of contact, he may instantly break the circuit by withdrawing his hand (and cautery tip) immediately on seeing the first darkening of tissue as the coagulation begins about the vessel.

Good cautery teamwork requires that the assistant be able to see the tip of the forceps clearly before he applies the cautery. He must also wait until the area of the surgical field about the forceps or clamp is dry. He may need to sponge the area himself. He should be certain that no metallic part of the coagulating clamp or forceps is making accidental contact with any part of the wound other than that to be coagulated. He must then hear the proper pitch of buzz that tells him that the coagulating (and not the cutting) current is activated. Then, and only then, should he permit himself to touch the forceps. He may touch

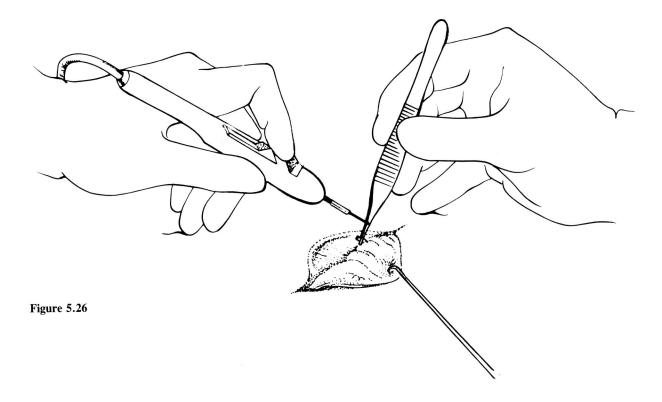

**Figure 5.26**

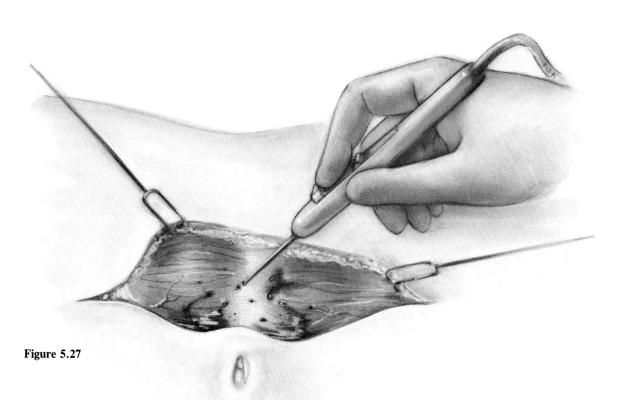

**Figure 5.27**

any part of the metal that is convenient, but he should touch lightly so as not to dislodge a delicate bite of the forceps on the tissues, and he should avoid blocking the surgeon's view of the operative field as he moves in to apply the cautery tip.

Above all, no assistant should ever apply the cautery unless he is first in a position to watch its effect on the tissues. He must not wait for verbal instruction from the surgeon to remove the current. Instead, he must learn the amount of current required to seal a vessel of given size, and withdraw the cautery tip the instant that point has been reached.

At times (Fig. 5.27), the cautery tip may be rapidly touched directly to the open ends of very small bleeding vessels, but this "dusting" technique may cause more necrosis than necessary if not executed with a light touch. In Figure 5.27, the tip of the activated cautery is moved quickly from one bleeding point to another where small vessels penetrate the fascia of the rectus muscle. The assistant should precede the cautery with suction or sponging to dry the surface and pinpoint the vessel openings. One should avoid placing the tip of the cautery directly on vessels that lie in the dermis of thin skin, on vessels near important nerves, or on any arterial branch at a point near a main parent artery that one wishes to preserve.

### Hemostasis in Bleeding Bone by Vessel Plugging

Pressures, sutures, clips, and the coagulating cautery are all rather unsatisfactory methods for stopping bleeding from the surface of bone. The cutting current will sometimes penetrate bone and work effectively to seal intra-osseous vessels, but bone damage may be excessive.

Bone wax may be used effectively to plug vessels in bleeding bone. In Figure 5.28 the convex surface of a Freer elevator is being used to apply the wax. Firm downward pressure forces the wax into the small bleeding bony canals. When the bleeding stops, all excess wax is carefully removed from the surface. It is helpful if the scrub nurse passes the wax with a small bolus stuck to the convex surface of a narrow and slightly curved elevator.

### Hemostasis With Drugs

**Vasoconstrictor drugs**

Vasoconstrictors such as epinephrine and norepinephrine are quite valuable in reducing blood loss. They may be injected into the skin and subcutaneous tissue before making an incision in any part of the body. The smooth muscle constriction in the vessel walls requires about 6 minutes to appear, but then it develops quite suddenly. It is best if the surgeon can inject the area and then busy himself for 5 to 10 minutes with another activity (such as scrubbing, prepping or draping the field, or marking out the incisions) before starting the operation.

The total dose of drug must be limited. If a concentration of 1:200,000 epinephrine in saline is used, one may safely inject 40 to 50 ml of this solution into an average-size adult weighing 70 kg. The anesthetist should be advised of the amount of vasoconstrictor used at the time of its injection.

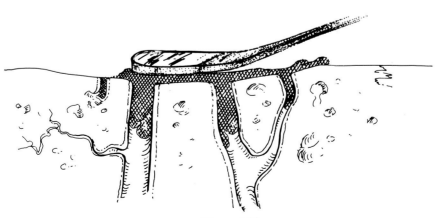

**Figure 5.28**

Epinephrine is of substantial value in reducing blood loss during operations under either local or general anesthesia. The reduction in bleeding is more impressive with local anesthesia than with general anesthesia, but quite effective with both. If an anesthetic such as bupivacaine (Marcaine, 0.25%) is added to the epinephrine, less general anesthetic will be required and the patient will have a substantial reduction in postoperative wound pain for 6 to 8 hours after surgery. Many surgeons fail to take advantage of these valuable vasoconstrictors when working on patients under general anesthesia.

Caution should be exercised in using regional injections of epinephrine within, or close to, the pedicles of flaps. The normal blood supply of that flap will be substantially reduced by both the vasoconstrictor drug and the surgical design of the operation that follows. Experimental studies clearly show that some flaps, that otherwise would have survived, will develop major areas of slough if vasoconstrictor drugs are also injected into the pedicle tissues.

With operations of long duration, it may be desirable to inject vasoconstrictor agents repeatedly, at intervals of approximately 90 minutes, to continue control of fine bleeding.

Cocaine solution (4% to 20%) is both a fine topical local anesthetic, and also a strong primary vasoconstrictor. It is particularly effective in reducing bleeding when applied to mucous membranes.

### Topical clotting agents

Thrombin solution, topical cellulose, and gel foam blocks are but some of the agents that may be of use when applied directly to oozing surfaces. These substances are primarily useful to arrest bleeding from multiple small bleeders that do not clot or retract in the normal manner. Such drugs should be held in contact with the bleeding surface by means of a moist pack for 5 to 10 minutes for most effective action.

Although these biologic hemostatic agents are designed to be absorbed by the body, it is best to remove any excess agent before closing the wound. Clot acceleration agents should never be used as the only means of controlling discrete arterial bleeding.

### Hemostasis by controlled systemic hypotension

Enderby and others, in the 1960s, pioneered in the deliberate reduction of systemic blood pressure during operations under general anesthesia in order to reduce bleeding and blood loss during surgery. In early experience, agents such as sodium nitroprusside were found to be somewhat dangerous, and postoperative bleeding was not uncommon when the blood pressures were brought back to normal levels. Today, the science of anesthesiology has brought increased safety to these techniques by better selection of patients, safer hypotensive agents, continuous monitoring of blood pressure with arterial lines, and the practice of providing gradual slow return of pressures to normal levels.

The wise surgeon will make use of hypotensive anesthesia. It will greatly reduce blood loss, provide a drier field in which to operate, and reduce total operating time. In many cases, operations may be performed without transfusion that otherwise would have required them. The risks of the patient developing hepatitis, AIDS, or some other viral infections from transfused blood are eliminated.

## Deliberate Embolism (Intravascular Occlusion of Regional Vessels)

Intra-arterial embolism and intravascular balloon tamponade offer two means of gaining control of bleeding by reducing the regional blood flow. This intravascular occlusion should be achieved during, or just prior to, the surgical operation.

### Intra-arterial embolism

The deliberate insertion of multiple absorbable emboli into the arterial tree may produce obstruction to the flow of blood in those vessels and allow the surgeon to resect a highly vascular or dangerous lesion with much less blood loss. Collateral circulation must be present and dependable in providing sufficient circulation to any remaining tissue to assure wound healing without ischemic gangrene.

To be effective, the emboli must become lodged in those arteries that dominantly supply the local area where the surgery is to be performed. In the case of AV malformations, the emboli must be placed in the vessels (shunts) of the malformation itself—and not merely in the more normal vessels that supply arterial blood to the area of pathology. The reduction in blood flow is most marked immediately after the emboli are injected. With time, collateral circulation will open other vessels and increase the blood flow to the area. If the emboli are absorbable (gel foam boluses), the embolized channels will also slowly regain patency. For these reasons, any definitive surgery or resection

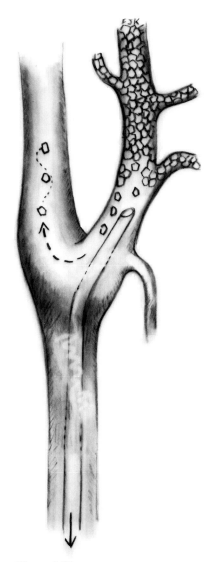

**Figure 5.29**

should be carried out as soon as practical after embolization in order to gain maximum control of hemostasis.

The cannula used to insert the emboli must be precisely placed in the perfusing arteries. This may be done by the radiologist, using fluoroscopic control, or catheters may be inserted by the surgeon at the outset of the operation, after he develops direct exposure of the vascular tree to be embolized.

The radiologist always runs some risk of dragging some of the inserted emboli back into the mainstream of a major artery when he withdraws the catheter. Figure 5.29 shows the radiologist's catheter (under fluoroscopic control) being withdrawn from the external carotid artery. Some of the emboli packed into the branches of the external carotid are being pulled back into the region of the carotid bulb along with the catheter tip. If these displaced straying emboli should then be carried into an undesirable vessel by the flow of blood, they may cause serious complications. In this case, they enter the internal carotid artery and produce hemiplegia. Several such tragic accidents have been reported in the medical literature. Although radiologists have developed great skill in placing catheters with selective embolization, this danger of straying emboli has not been eliminated.

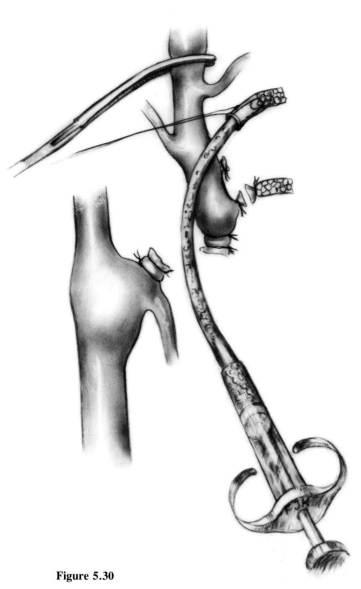

**Figure 5.30**

The risk of accidental hemiplegia may be completely avoided if the surgeon will do his own embolization, especially when operating on the head and neck. Figure 5.30 shows a safer method of suture ligation and division of the branches of the external carotid artery before insertion of the cannula and the packing of gel foam pledgets into those selected for embolization. With this system, there is no way for emboli to accidently enter the internal carotid artery. An attempt is made to pack individually, each of the feeder arteries leading into the malformation with gel foam pledgets soaked in thrombin. A small high-pressure syringe is used to force the emboli through the narrow lumen of an intracath catheter. As the vessel is filled, the catheter is slowly withdrawn. The artery, once packed throughout its entire length, is then ligated.

Embolism will greatly reduce bleeding in the removal of lesions such as arteriovenous fistulae and other highly vascular hamartomas.

### Intravascular balloon tamponade

Vascular surgeons are sometimes forced to control bleeding from major vessels such as the aorta while in the act of repairing these structures. Partial clamping or temporary complete cross-clamping of a large opened vessel may be needed to arrest exsanguinating hemorrhage. When the injury is proximal to the renal arteries (in the case of an aorta), a shunt may be needed to maintain flow around the area while the repair is in progress.

In a few instances, the insertion and inflation of a balloon on a catheter within the lumen of the artery may allow control of bleeding while the repair of the artery is completed. The details of these, occasionally needed, special techniques of hemostasis are described in detail in texts on vascular surgery.

## Removing Blood and Clots From Surgical Wounds

Once active bleeding has been controlled, the surgeon will want to remove any liquid or clotted blood that occupies the dependent recesses of the field. Such spilled blood not only obstructs vision but, if left in a wound, will produce a damaging effect that will delay the healing of tissues.

The surgeon removes this blood in three common ways: by sponging, suction, or irrigation.

## Sponging

Although sponging is a simple technique, it is often done badly by surgeons or their assistants. James Barrett Brown of Barnes Hospital in St. Louis was known to observe that you could judge the quality of a surgeon, in part, by the way he sponged a wound.

Gauze sponges are designed to absorb blood and fluid. Their absorptive qualities will draw up fluid much like a wick, but clots adhere to tissue and require a different action. If an assistant wishes to remove clotted blood from a wound, he must first press the sponge firmly against it and then use a slight pinching or grasping motion of his fingers (Fig. 5.31) to lift the clot away from the wound. His purpose should be to remove all of the clot in a single motion, with as little damage (caused by rubbing the tissue with the dry gauze) to the wound as possible. He should avoid ineffective and time-consuming repeated dabbing at the wound with his sponge. Any heavy rubbing of the wound should be avoided. When the offending blood is still liquid, a gentle blotting action with the sponge is all that is required. The sponging motion of the surgical assistant should be rapid and timed to occur between movements of the surgeon so that the field is cleanest at the moment just before the setting of the first throw of a knot, the touch of the cautery, or the use of the knife or needle. These are moments when details within the wound should be most clearly seen.

Sponges are expensive and should not be discarded until their absorptive surfaces are exhausted. Once soaked, they should promptly be removed from the field. If the operation demands a sponge count, be careful that sponges do not get tucked beneath drapes or placed in other obscure locations. When large body cavities are opened, all packs and sponges should be tagged to avoid their loss in some recess of the wound.

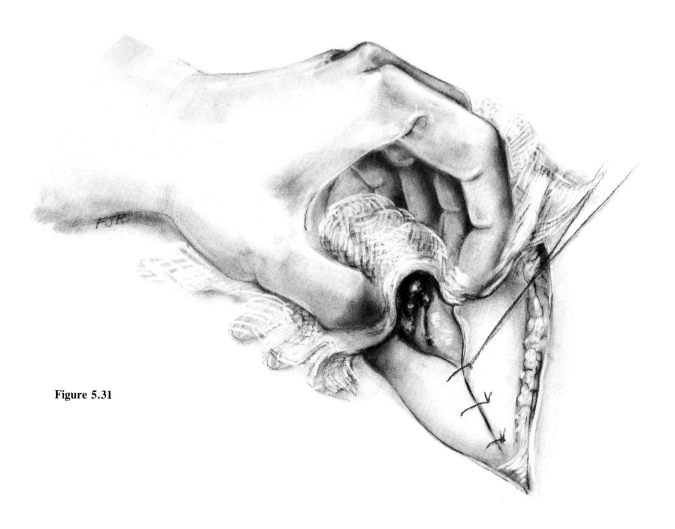

**Figure 5.31**

### Suction

The suction cannula, improperly used, is an instrument of the devil! It is noisy and traumatic to tissue. It increases blood loss and sometimes obstructs the vision of the surgeon.

Despite these drawbacks, suction plays a valuable role in surgery. Its function is to give the surgeon precise visibility of a particular part of the wound at a particular instant in time. The tip of the suction cannula should hover near the edge of the surgeon's knife (Fig. 5.32). Note that the assistant rests the little finger of his left-hand on the patient to improve his control of the tip of the cannula. It should be rapidly moved to lightly brush the deepest portion of the area being dissected. When working in tight areas or seeking a single bleeder, the assistant should hold the sucker in his fingertips. The surgeon's knife or scissors may be lightly touched, but should not be heavily bumped or displaced by its tip. Suction is needed precisely at the point of dissection or clamping, and not at some remote portion of the wound.

Wound suction is a job for the first assistant. He should be certain that neither the sucker nor his hand occupies the line of vision between the surgeon's eye and the point of dissection. If he keeps the tip moving quickly back and forth, visibility will not be compromised. A very small diameter suction tip is needed in narrow recesses or small wounds. If tissues are very delicate or fragile (as about the eyelids), the suction force (valve on vacuum at the wall) should be reduced. The small vent on many suction tips may also be left open to get more gentle suction. Occlusion of this opening will appropriately vary the suction force at the tip. At times a bit of gauze may be draped over the tip of the sucker further to reduce the suction force.

If the suction cannula becomes blocked, the assistant should quickly remove the tip from the tubing to be certain that the latter is still patent. Saline should be flushed through the tip and tubing at intervals to clean it of blood clots (Fig. 5.33). A rubber bulb (asepto) syringe and short segment of rubber tubing may help open a balky cannula and save both expense and nursing time.

When the operative field is relatively dry and suction is not required, the assistant or nurse should kink or clamp off the tubing to reduce the noise level. A quiet operating room improves the quality of surgery!

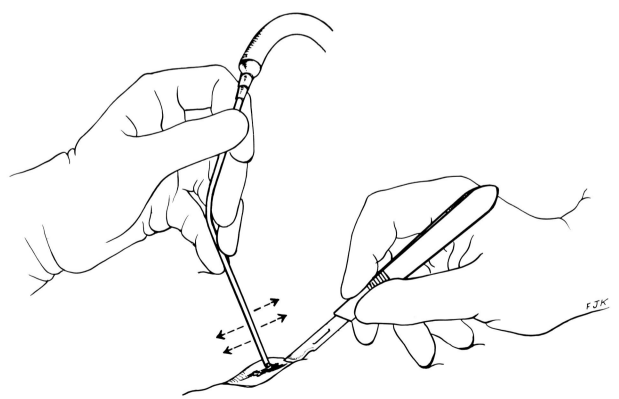

**Figure 5.32**

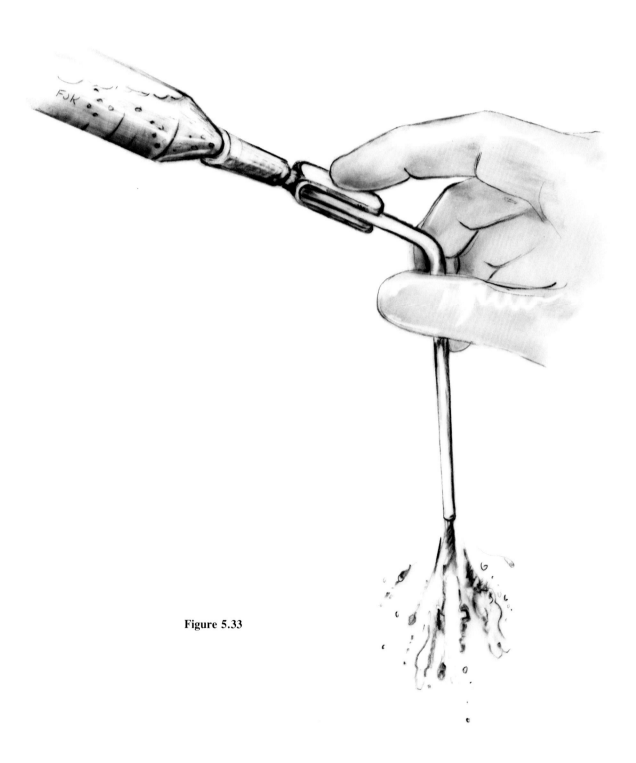

**Figure 5.33**

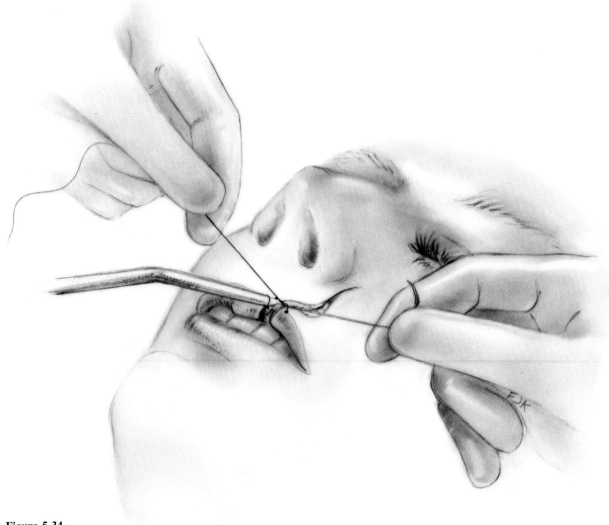

**Figure 5.34**

When sutures are being placed and tied, suction may be used to remove all blood from the tissue in the area to be sutured. This should be done just before the surgeon inserts the needle. A few moments later, the suction again will be of value to remove any blood from the suture just before he sets the tension on the first loop of his knot (Fig. 5.34). Needle insertion and knot setting should be done when the wound is free of all blood and clots, and maximum visibility is provided.

## Irrigation

### Physiologic saline

Wound irrigation with physiologic saline has several purposes. It removes blood, clots, and any detached tissue. It reduces the bacterial count and removes free cancer cells that might otherwise implant in the wound as grafts. It moistens tissues.

Irrigation with distilled water has also been used to produce osmotic forces that will lyse any free cancer cells and thus further reduce the chance that they seed the wound with new tumors.

Wounds resulting from gross trauma may contain large quantities of soil particles, grease, and other foreign bodies. Removal of some of these substances may require irrigation with a jet of fluid under moderate pressure. Such "pressure jet" irrigations should not be directed into deep tissue planes as they may produce interstitial emphysema and carry particles into deeper recesses and tissue planes that are well beyond the original wound.

Most wound irrigation is best done with a rubber bulb syringe or by use of a gravity-drip system of modest height (3 feet). A collecting basin is placed along the most dependent margin of the wound, the skin edges are lifted to create a *well*, and the saline is injected in short bursts, starting first in the most superior recesses of the wound. The surgeon in Figure 5.35 is using his gloved finger to open recesses, loosen adherent clots, and elevate the deeper tissues to improve the washing mechanics of the stream. Some of the irrigating solution may then be used to clean blood

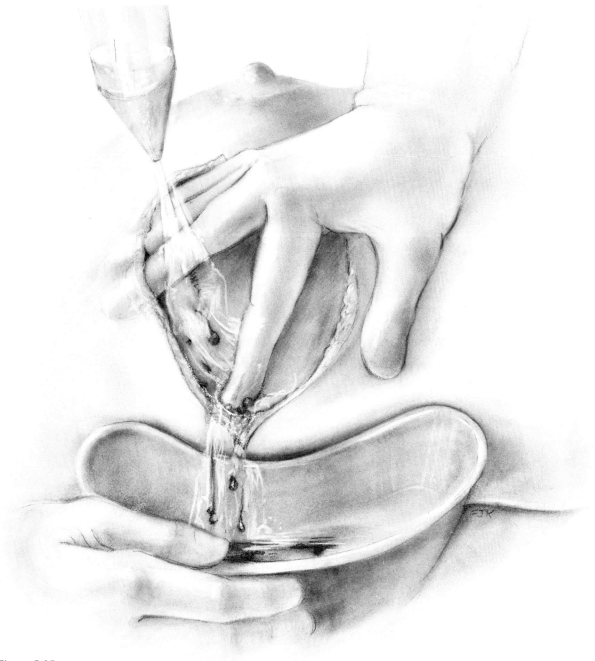

**Figure 5.35**

from the external surfaces of the skin. Wound irrigations of this type should be repeated at intervals throughout long operations.

Copious irrigation with physiologic saline is correlated with significant reductions in wound infection rates of post-traumatic injuries.

### Topical antibiotic solutions

Surgeons periodically become enthusiastic about antibiotic irrigation as a further method of reducing postoperative wound infection rates. This concept has received considerable support from experimental studies. However, the bactericidal qualities of any antibiotic solution must be balanced against any osmotic or chemical qualities that will damage the normal cells within the wound.

On the basis of a number of experimental studies, the author has used bacitracin solution as a wound irrigant since 1974 with a resulting minimal wound infection rate and no clinical evidence of reduction in rate or quality of wound healing. This solution may be used even on the surface of the brain or in the conjunctival sac with no evidence of deleterious effects.

# 6
## Suturing Wounds

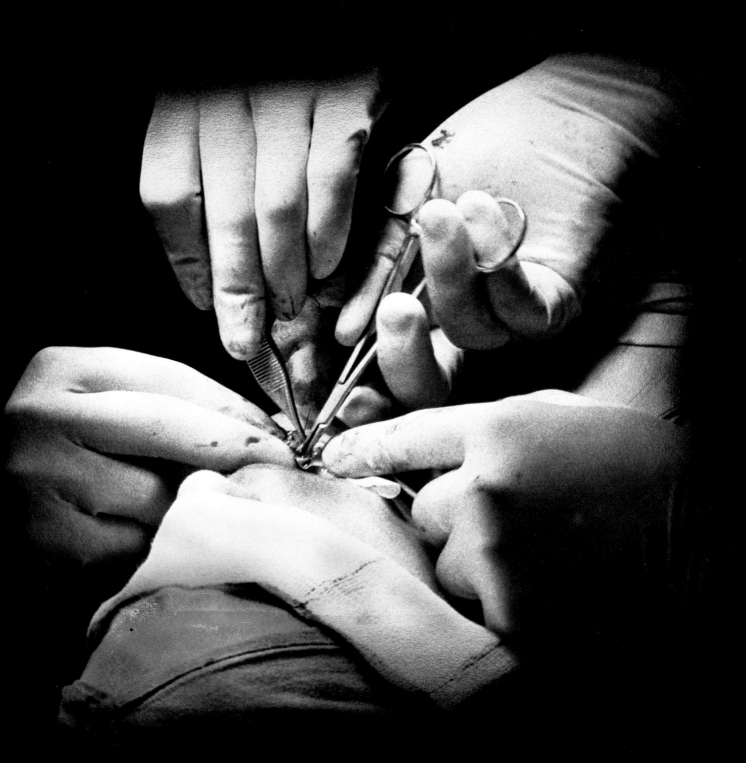

# 6
## Suturing Wounds

# Needles and Sutures

### Handheld Needles

Some large surgical needles are designed to be held and passed with the fingers. Most of these are straight needles that are long enough to be useful in transfixing a large bite of tissue. The three-sided cutting points of Keith needles and the round, noncutting fine intestinal needles are examples of finger-held needles. One convenient use of the long straight cutting needle is in the joining together of two skin grafts. In Figure 6.1 a straight needle is used to evert the overlapping remaining edges of two skin grafts that are being joined together. The grafts were first sutured to the margins of the defect with running continuous sutures. The surgeon now wants to join the two thin grafts to one another to complete wound closure. He pleats the graft edges back and forth over the slowly advancing straight needle. The technique allows 7 or 8 bites before pulling the needle through and is much more rapid than doing the same job with a curved needle. Here the tissue is put on the needle—not the needle on the tissue. When this basting stitch is secured at each end, an excellent approximation of the graft results. This particular straight needle has a cutting tip and an eye that permits it to be hand-threaded. Many straight needles are made with swaged-on suture material.

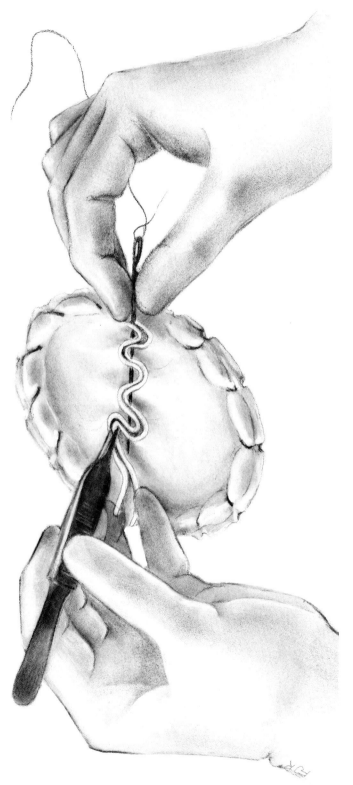

**Figure 6.1**

## Pie-Crust Suturing of Skin Grafts

At the circular margin of the defect shown in Figure 6.2, a split thickness graft has been sutured with a pie-crust method, using a running suture to snug the graft into contact with the vertical raw edges of the surrounding skin. The skin graft was first placed over the defect with its margins slightly overlapping the edge. A curved needle is used to place each bite, first going through the skin graft, then through the skin margin, and out again through the overlapping edge of the graft (Fig. 6.2, *inset*). This suture holds the graft nicely tucked down to seal all raw surfaces of the wound, including the vertical section of the elevated skin edge. This prevents graft bridging and hematoma collection. It is an excellent and rapid method of applying large split-thickness skin grafts to burn wounds. Any excess overlapping skin is then trimmed away with scissors. The sutures are removed at the first postoperative dressing, and final trimming of all skin graft overlap is done at that time.

## Selection of Needles and Needle Holders

Smaller needles are almost always passed with the aid of needle-holding clamps. The box-locked jaws of needle holders are short, wide, and strong enough to prevent turning of the needle when it encounters dense tissue. When needle holders are used for tying sutures, it is helpful if their jaws have smooth surfaces. This prevents jaw serrations from weakening the suture material and reduces the tendency of fine suture materials to slip out of the jaw when being tied.

Needles and sutures should be chosen appropriately for the task required. Cutting needles should always be used to sew the skin, but round, taper-point needles are better for repairing a lacerated liver or the walls of large or small bowel or blood vessels. When small suture bites are required or delicate, thin tissues are sewn, small needles and fine suture materials are needed. These same fine materials may be totally inappropriate for large, tougher tissues that must be sutured under considerable tension.

Needles that are individually hand-sharpened are consistently sharper than those sharpened by machines during production. Hand sharpening adds considerable extra expense and these precision needle tips should not be requested when the tissues to be sutured do not require them.

Swaged-on suture material improves the ease of passage of the needle and its thread, but the hand-threaded needle continues to serve well (and economically) in many surgical situations.

Recently, lasers have been used to make tiny holes in the base of fine needles. The suture material end is then fixed into this hole to improve the swage. Even so, the needle diameters remain three times the diameters of the attached suture material.

Surgeons and nurses must remain cost-conscious and not automatically request the most expensive item for all occasions. The ideal suture of the future will come from a technology that allows us to stiffen and sharpen the tip of an inert and flexible strand of suture material. Perhaps we can "metallize" the tip of a strand of silk or nylon—or coat it with a cone of sharpened glass!

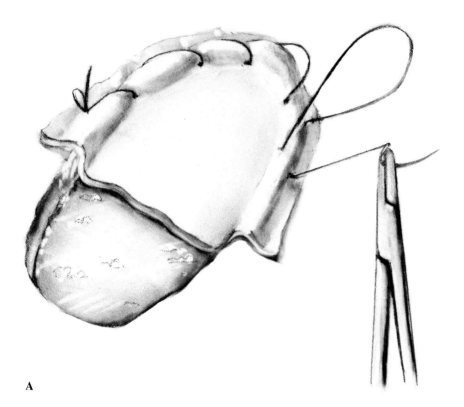

A

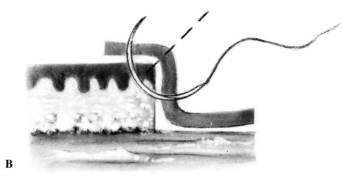

B

Figure 6.2

## Use of the Needle Holder

The surgeon should receive the needle holder in the palm of his dominant hand. The scrub nurse should firmly smack it against his glove so that he can feel the handle without shifting his eyes from the brightly lighted operative field to the darker area of the Mayo instrument stand. Frequent pupillary constriction and dilation can add to eye fatigue.

The tip of the needle should always point toward the ceiling of the operating room and then tilt toward the surgeon, as his hand opens, as shown in Figure 6.3. The nurse should have the straightened suture trailing loosely over the back of her wrist. The jaws of the needle holder should grasp the needle quite close to its swaged butt. This position gives the surgeon maximum length of needle shaft to engage the tissue. The handle of the needle holder should make contact with the surgeon's palm with a firm "pop" so that he knows to close his hand without taking his eyes from the surgical field.

In this fashion, the surgeon takes the handle of the needle holder with no risk of including the trailing suture material in his grasp. As he moves the needle holder into position for use, the trailing length of the suture material glides over the nurse's wrist. The surgeon should feel no sensation of pulling or catching of the suture against any resistance that might risk breaking it. The nurse should never try to feed the suture directly to the surgeon as it leaves the suture package while she is still holding the container. She should clear the suture from the packet and straighten its bends and curls with a firm tug before the surgeon reaches for it. The surgeon should indicate his choice of needle and suture size well in advance of needing

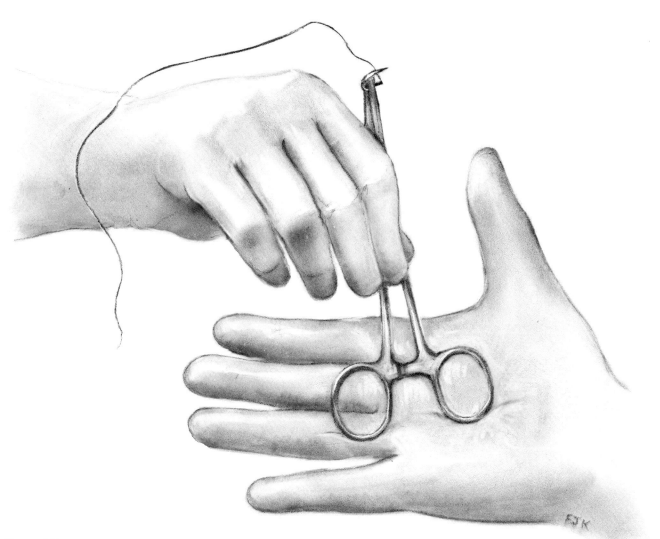

**Figure 6.3**

it, but if he fails to do so it is the nurse's responsibility to request this information in good time.

The surgeon will usually have a pair of forceps (Fig. 6.4) or a skin hook (Fig. 6.5) in his nondominant hand to stabilize the tissue as he passes his needle. They are used to brace the skin as the tip of the needle emerges on the "exit" side of an incision during closure. The sharp prongs of the forceps or hook are "set" into the tissue only when necessary to avoid slipping. More complete use of these instruments is

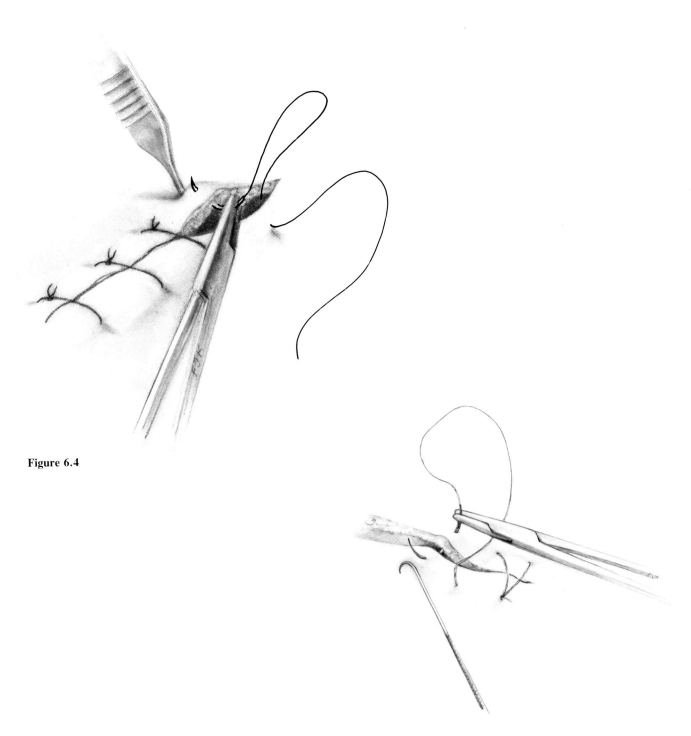

**Figure 6.4**

**Figure 6.5**

illustrated in Chapter 3. When sewing delicate tissues such as skin of the face, the surgeon can minimize tissue damage if he uses only his gloved finger or a folded sponge (Figs. 6.6 and 6.7) to fix the target skin in place as the needle is passed.

In Fig. 6.6 the sponge holds the skin margin down and protects the surgeon's fingertips. Once the needle tip has emerged through the skin and into the sponge, the sponge is lifted (Fig. 6.7), and the needle is grasped by the needle holder and withdrawn.

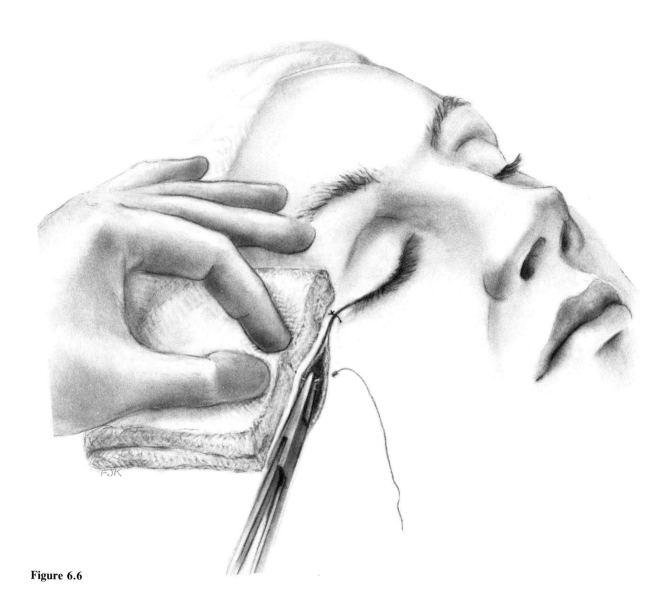

**Figure 6.6**

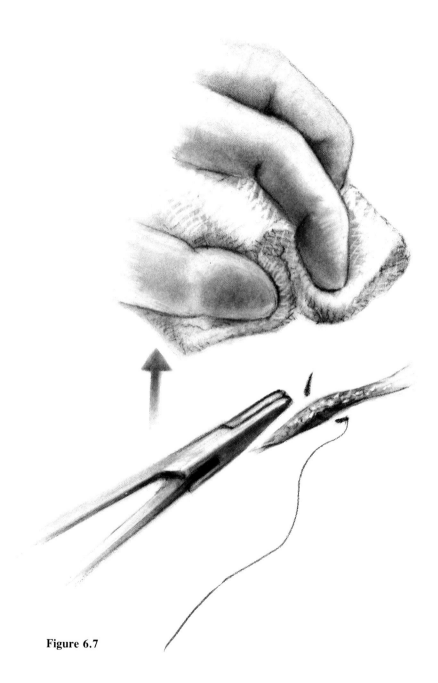

**Figure 6.7**

## Suturing Skin

### Inserting the Needle

In placing the initial bite with the needle, the surgeon will presupinate his wrist to cock his hand into a strong position for driving the needle through the skin (Fig. 6.8). The one ring of the needle holder rests against the palm of the hand. In most instances, the needle is pushed through the tissues without placing the fingers or thumb in the needle holder rings. The flexed index finger presses the tip of the needle vertically downward, and a strong supination motion of the wrist forces the needle through the tissue as the nose of the needle holder inscribes a small half-circle that matches the curve of the needle. To produce this supination, the surgeon's little and ring fingers force one ring of the needle holder downward as the other is pushed upward by the base of the thumb where it grips the ring against the palm. The motion of rotation is more efficient if the long axis of the needle holder is held so that it approximates a continuation of the axis of the radius of the forearm.

The needle may be passed with a single motion through one or both sides of the wound, depending on the length of the needle, the thickness of the skin, and the tension separating the two sides of the wound.

### Obtaining Ideal Skin Approximation

Whenever a skin edge is sutured with a simple full-thickness cuticular suture, the passage of the needle should include deep dermis that is further removed from the cut margin of the skin than is the entrance or exit point of the suture through the epidermis. This gives the tied suture a somewhat pyramidal shape when viewed in cross-section (Fig. 6.9) and improves dermal approximation. The mild vertical lifting of the entire suture line that results is sometimes called the "Halsted roll." The tendency of the approximated tissues to contract downward with postoperative healing and produce a depression is partially off-set by starting the healing from this initial slightly elevated position of the approximated skin edges.

The skin hook or toothed forceps is helpful in everting the skin edges as the surgeon sets the tip of the needle so that it will follow the desired direction in its passage through the dermis.

On the second side of the incision, the surgeon may use the tip of his needle as in Figure 6.10 to engage the dermis and aid the forceps in rolling out the skin margin. The dermis is first everted with the needle tip. It is then grasped beneath the level of the epidermis with the forceps before resetting the tip of the needle and pressing it out through that skin margin (Fig. 6.11). The surgeon will see improvement in the final healing and smoothness of cutaneous scars if he will give attention to such details in suturing. After a little practice such points of technique become second nature.

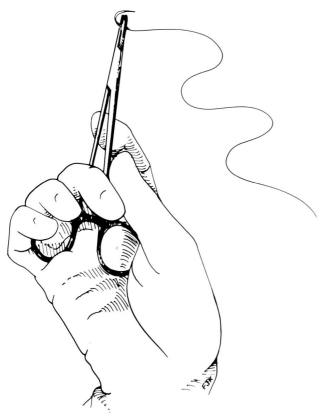

**Figure 6.8**

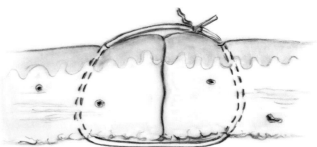

**Figure 6.9**

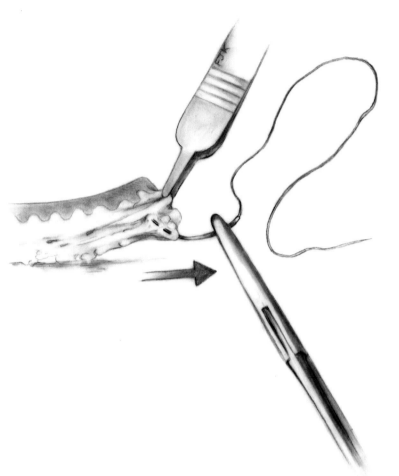

**Figure 6.10**

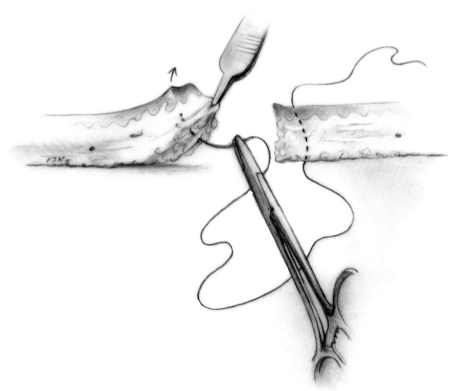

**Figure 6.11**

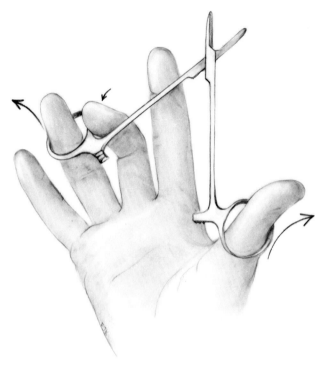

**Figure 6.12**

### Role of the Assistant

When the point of the needle emerges from the tissue, it may be grasped by an assistant who simply fixes it in position with a second needle holder until the surgeon can release his instrument. This he does by separating the rings and releasing the ratchet of his needle holder (Fig. 6.12). By extending and rotating his thumb, that ring is pushed away from his palm. At the same time, the flexing of the distal joints of his index, long, and ring fingers help force the other ring (and handle) of the needle holder back toward the palm—thus disengaging the teeth of the ratchet.

If the surgeon is tying the knots, the assistant will return the needle to him and prepare to cut the suture. If the assistant is tying the knots, the surgeon will leave the needle with the assistant and return his needle holder to the scrub nurse in exchange for another with the next needle and suture already mounted. In this case, after the suture is cut, the assistant returns the first needle and remaining length of suture to the scrub nurse. She will continue to reuse each suture until its length becomes too short for easy tying. Details of knot tying by hand are discussed in Chapter 5.

### Tying Knots With the Needle Holder

It is often useful to tie knots with a needle holder as skin or other tissues are being sutured. This may speed the closure and conserve suture material by allowing many sutures to be obtained from a single strand of suture material with its swaged-on needle. Significant cost savings will result.

Either the surgeon or his assistant may do the actual tying with a needle holder. In the latter case, the assistant uses a second smooth-jawed needle holder with which he first grasps the needle tip (Fig. 6.13) as it emerges through the skin on the side of exit. The surgeon releases his bite, (Fig. 6.14) and the assistant rotates the needle sufficiently to withdraw it from the skin (Fig. 6.15). He then grasps the needle near the midportion of its shaft between the tips of the

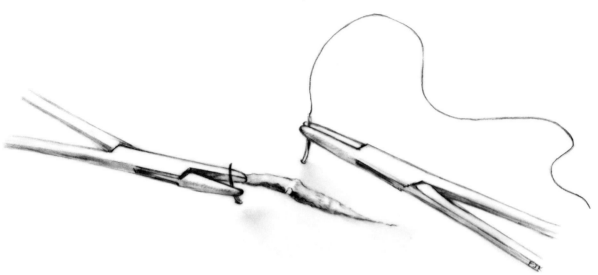

**Figure 6.13**

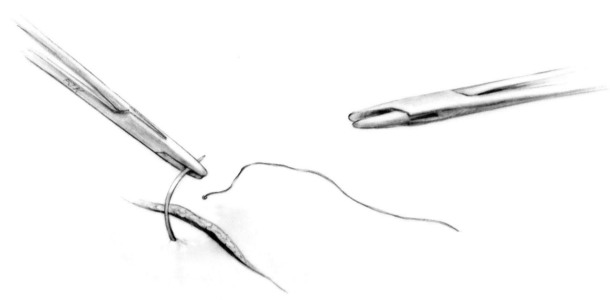

**Figure 6.14**

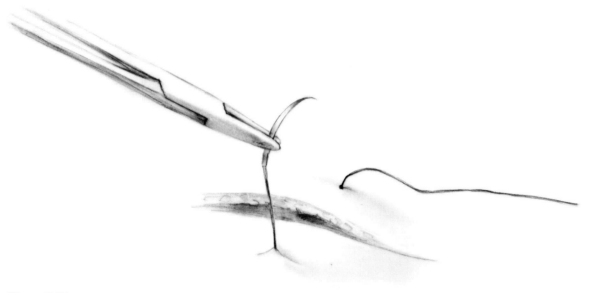

**Figure 6.15**

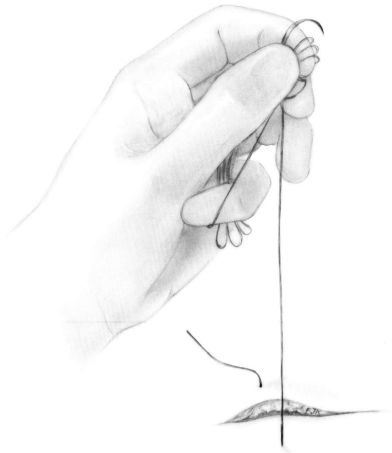

**Figure 6.16**

thumb and index finger of his nondominant hand. A rapid rotating action of his wrist allows him to pull the suture material through the tissue and pleat it in his fingers (Fig. 6.16) until only a 1- to 2-inch short end remains and most of the suture is plicated in several loops in the fingers and palm of his left hand. He then throws a loop of the long end of the suture over the tip of his needle holder and grasps the remaining short end. This is pulled down, and the knot is laid flat and tightened. When the knot tension and skin edge approximation are ideal, the knot is squared by throwing a second loop in the suture material (Fig. 6.17A) over the tip of the needle holder. This loop is flipped in the opposite direction from the first so that the knot will be squared. As several knots are added

for security, the assistant will use a slight flipping action with the tip of the needle holder to loosen the suture material as it slides down the shaft of the needle holder. This motion keeps the suture material from dropping into the hinge of the box lock and getting caught there with each throw. The assistant then holds up the short end of the suture with the needle holder alongside the long end in his nondominant hand, and the suture is cut (Fig. 6.17B).

Throughout this process, the assistant has retained the needle securely between the thumb and index fingers of his left hand. He now drops the pleated excess suture material and clamps his needle holder on the needle. He returns both to the scrub nurse or surgeon.

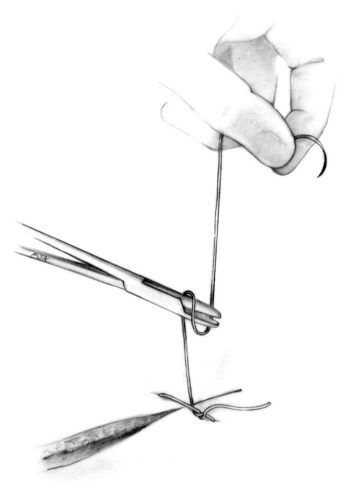

**Figure 6.17A**

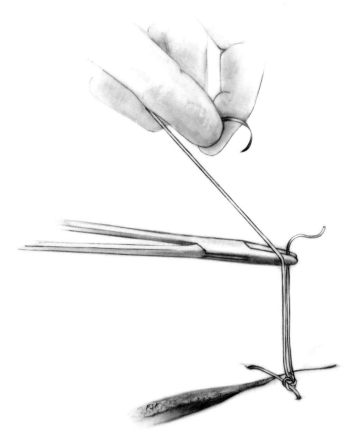

**Figure 6.17B**

If the surgeon is using his own needle holder to tie skin sutures, the assistant only "fixes the needle" for him. In fixing a needle for the surgeon, the assistant first clamps the emerging needle with his needle holder just behind the tip—at a point that will not damage the delicate needle tip. He then rotates the needle around the arc of its curve so that roughly 80% of the needle emerges from the skin. *He does not want the entire needle to come free from the skin!* If the needle comes free (and becomes airborne), it will be difficult to hold it steady and transfer it quickly back into the surgeon's needle holder. If, however, the end of the needle remains clamped in the assistant's needle holder, and the base is still fixed in the skin, it becomes a simple matter for the surgeon to recover the needle with his own needle holder (Fig. 6.18). He then transfers the needle to his left hand as he begins an instrument tie.

If the suture is long, the surgeon pinches the needle with his left thumb and index finger, plicates the long end of the suture (Fig. 6.16), ties the knots with his needle holder, and holds up the ends for the assistant to cut. He then drops the several loops of plicated suture and grasps the needle (still held in his left thumb and index pinch) with the needle holder in a position ready for him to take his next stitch.

## Subcuticular Sutures

### When to Use—or Not Use

Some incisions will heal with finer scars if subcuticular sutures are used before the skin sutures are applied. This deep row of sutures will reduce the dead space, lower the tension on skin sutures needed for fine approximation of skin margins, and allow earlier removal of skin sutures so as to avoid hatchmarking.

*Subcuticular sutures should never be placed in the superficial dermis.* To do so invites suture extrusion, infection, lumpy or irregular healing, and dissatisfied patients. Unless the dermis is very thick (as with the skin of the back), it should never be included in the bite of a subcuticular suture.

### Placing the Knots Deep

Problems with subcuticular sutures will be reduced if care is taken always to bury the knot at the deepest point of the suture loop. The surgeon should learn a definite technique of suturing that allows knot burial with minimal trauma. In Figure 6.19A the surgeon has first placed the needle in the subcutaneous fascia so as to include a small amount of the deep

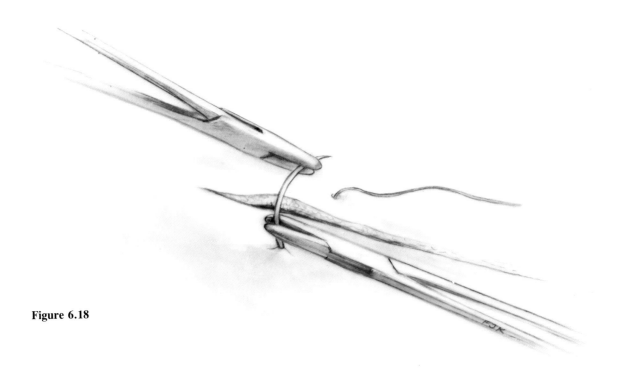

**Figure 6.18**

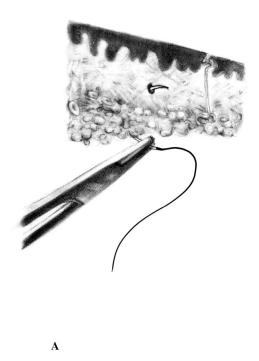

**A**

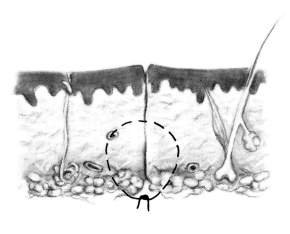

**B**

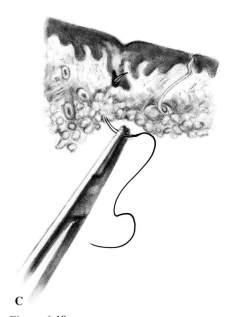

**C**

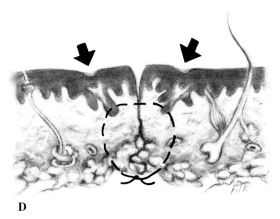

**D**

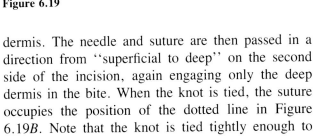

**Figure 6.19**

dermis. The needle and suture are then passed in a direction from "superficial to deep" on the second side of the incision, again engaging only the deep dermis in the bite. When the knot is tied, the suture occupies the position of the dotted line in Figure 6.19*B*. Note that the knot is tied tightly enough to

bring the tissues together, but not so tight as to cause ischemic necrosis. The upper dermis is nicely opposed and slightly elevated above the surrounding skin surface. The incision is now ready for a very fine cuticular suture to ensure vertical alignment of the epidermis during the postoperative period.

### Errors in Placing Subcuticular Sutures

In Figure 6.19*C* the operator is placing his needle so that it catches too much of the upper dermis. Figure 6.19*D* shows the result of this more superficial bite. When this error has occurred, the external surface of the skin is usually dimpled on either side of the incision, and the epidermis may be held in a slightly separated position when the knot is tied. In his efforts to improve any apparent imperfect approximation of the skin, the surgeon will be tempted to tie the knots in his cuticular sutures too tightly and produce vascular obstruction, cell death, and delayed healing. If that error is repeated with the placement of each stitch, the accumulated damage becomes substantial.

Subcuticular sutures are most valuable in closing skin in parts of the body with thick dermal layers, or when the skin is firmly attached to strong subdermal fascia that will hold sutures well. They are especially useful when there is significant tension on the closure.

When the dermis is thin, the superficial subcuticular suture should be avoided. When there is little tension on the closure, the subcuticular suture line may not be needed. A good surgeon will individualize his skin closure techniques, considering the exact anatomy of the skin, the tension on closure, and the expected postoperative movements of that particular incision.

### Placing Subcuticular Sutures With Minimal Trauma

The ideal placement of a subcuticular suture should involve minimum handling of the skin with crushing instruments. A skin hook will provide an excellent combination of control and eversion of the skin edges with little injury to the skin itself. The hook tip is fixed by "setting" it into the tissue by pressure against the tip of the index finger. This firmly clamps the skin edge, allowing the surgeon to lift and evert it.

Figure 6.20 shows how the operator uses his

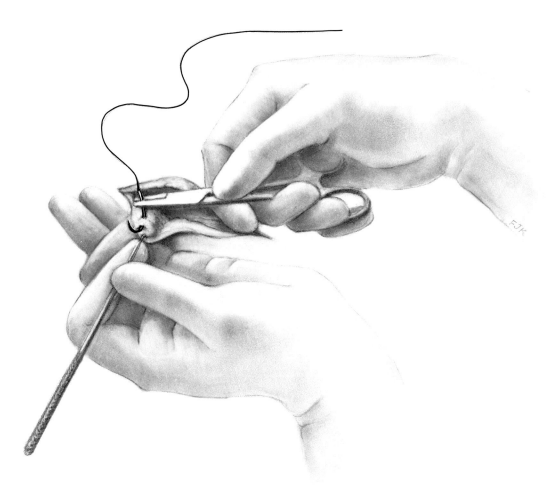

**Figure 6.20**

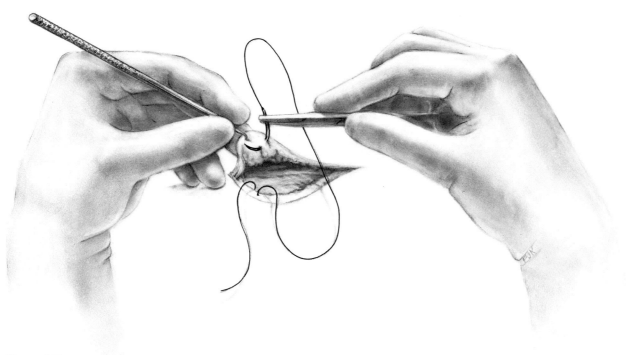

**Figure 6.21**

nondominant hand as the first bite of a subcuticular suture (with a buried knot) is placed. His thumb and index finger control the hook. He is using the tip of his left long finger to monitor the depth of bite of the needle. Note that the long axis of the needle is at about a 45° angle with the edge of the skin.

The needle holder has passed the needle in a direction from deep to superficial, picking up some of the firm subdermal fascia. The needle also travels a few millimeters laterally before emerging at the more superficial point.

In Figure 6.21 the needle has been withdrawn from the tissue on the near side of the incision and the hook has been shifted to fix and evert the opposite edge of the wound (note the resting of the ring and little fingers of the hook-holding hand against the skin of the patient to steady and relax that hand). Here the hook tip works as a partner with the tip of the left long finger to evert and secure the skin margin. The needle is now being placed, using a bite that travels from superficial to deep. Once more the needle is inserted at a 45° angle so that it travels a horizontal distance through the dermis that equals the vertical

distance of the needle path in the deep-to-superficial bite that was taken on the first side of the incision (Fig. 6.20). Note again that, when this suture is tied, the knot will lie at the deepest part of the suture loop, and some degree of both vertical and horizontal approximation of the deep tissues on the two sides of the wound will have been obtained.

## Long-Term Fate of Subcuticular Nylon

Fine nylon has proved to be an effective material for subcuticular sutures. Yet even nylon should be avoided unless the skin is thick enough to allow it to be placed deeply. Sutures of 5-0 or 4-0 clear nylon should be spaced at least 10 mm apart, and their ends should be cut on the knot. Clear nylon does not leave a dark discoloration that will later show through skin. Nylon buried in human tissue slowly breaks down over a two-year period into two simple molecules that are both mildly bacteriostatic.

# The Running Intradermal Pull-Out Suture

### Advantages

One of the most valuable sutures for closing human skin is the running intradermal pull-out suture. Since this suture will be removed postoperatively and cause no troublesome late problems of extrusion or infection, it may be placed in the dermis close to the skin surface. When prolene or nylon is used as an intradermal pull-out to close skin under some tension, it may be left in place for weeks without causing significant inflammatory reactions. When this tension is significant, delayed suture removal may be prudent. In these circumstances, use of the intradermal pull-out suture avoids producing the hatchmark scars that are commonly caused by other types of skin sutures.

This simple suture technique provides both subcuticular and cuticular layer closure, since the bites may grasp the strong dermal layer in their central portions and still enter and exit the tissue so superficially that they also provide excellent epidermal approximation.

The intradermal pull-out suture requires a strong suture material that has a very low coefficient of friction. Prolene or nylon will serve well. Prolene is somewhat easier to remove but is also somewhat more brittle than nylon. Both cause minimal tissue reactivity. One should *not* use a suture material such as Novafil® that will give or lengthen under tension. If such a material is used, postoperative edema and movements will stretch the suture and loosen the suture line. Approximation will be lost as the material does not contract back to its original length.

And ideal suture material would lengthen slightly in response to wound edema, but then shorten to its *original length* as the edema subsides.

### Technique of Placing

This type of suture must be placed and tied, with great care. A single interrupted suture is first placed as shown in the upper inset in Figure 6.22. Here a chest incision is being closed following the removal of a rib bone graft. The closure starts at the inferior end of the wound. Several knots are tied and a clamp is attached to the short end so that the assistant might give countertraction as the suturing continues. The needle then re-enters the skin several millimeters further down along one side and emerges through the dermis quite close to the dermal-epidermal junction. The needle then advances along the incision as it is crossed back and forth to engage corresponding points along the two skin edges. At each point a substantial bite is taken (*upper inset* in Fig. 6.22) so that the suture will encompass several millimeters of stout dermis before reemerging at the dermal-epidermal junction. The surgeon may avoid forceps damage by using the back of his skin hook to atraumatically brace the skin as the needle is pushed through the dermis. Although the needle tip enters and exits the cut surface of the skin margin superficially (at the epidermal-dermal junction), each bite is angled downward as the needle is pushed in, allowing the tip, at the midpoint of its bite, to engage a deep and stout portion of the reticular dermis, well back from the cut margins of the skin. This angling of the needle is essential if the suture is to provide both secure closure and excellent approximation of the superficial skin margins.

As the sewing continues, each new bite in tissue in the opposite side of the incision begins exactly across from the exit point of the needle from the first side. If one places this point of needle entry either too far back or too far forward, the skin margins will gape or buckle as the suture is tightened and tied. On reaching the end of the incision, the needle is allowed to emerge through the skin epidermis. It is then reversed and passed through both skin edges. The loop and long end are pulled to tighten the suture and bring the skin edges firmly together. While this tension is held, the needle end of the suture is looped around the tip of the needle holder and tied to the prolene loop as shown in the lower inset of Figure 6.22.

After 7 to 14 days, the suture may be removed by cutting the suture loop at each end of the incision. The knot is then cut off of one end, and the other knot is used to pull out the suture slowly from one end. The suture should slide easily if the original bites were properly placed. Should the prolene or nylon become stuck, the elastic band technique described in the section in Chapter 7 on ''Suture Removal'' should be used.

The intradermal pull-out suture can be used in any part of the body. The avoidance of permanent stitch marks and easy painless removal of the suture make it very popular with patients. Although this suture should be placed very carefully and in an unhurried manner, it will usually save time as it replaces two rows of suture that might otherwise be required.

If there is any minor irregularity of epidermal approximation after the pull-out suture is tied, paper tape or fine 6-0 silk sutures can be added in spots where needed.

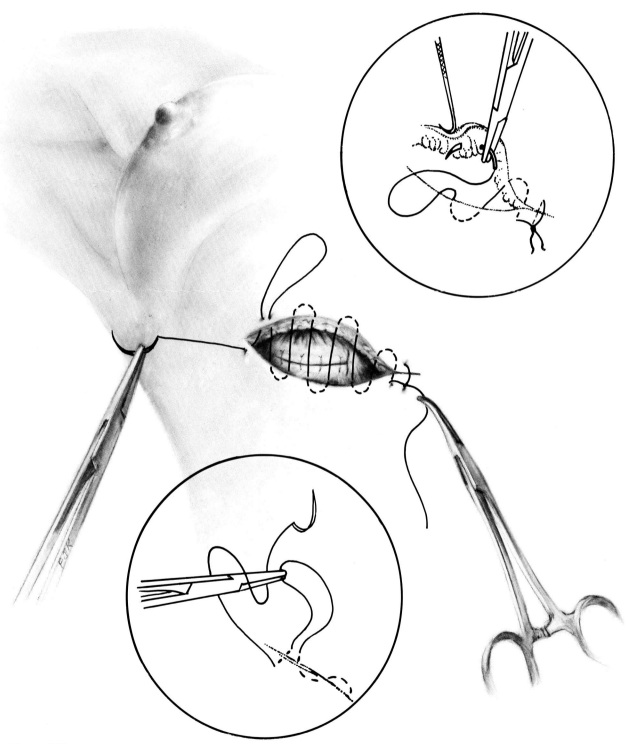

**Figure 6.22**

We have learned that even many facial scars may be improved by selective use of the intradermal pull-out suture. Surgeons of all specialties would do well to make more use of this skin closure method. It should replace the running cuticular suture that is still used for many closures. Patients who observe a neat skin closure often conclude that the "inside" suturing by their surgeon was done with equal care!

## Running Cuticular Suture

### Advantages and Disadvantages

The running cuticular suture has long been a favorite of surgeons. It is an easy and rapid method of skin closure. It requires minimal technical skill, and the suture is readily removed, postoperatively.

On the negative side, a running suture does not approximate skin as accurately as do either interrupted or properly placed intradermal sutures. It also tends to cause ischemia of the skin margins. With any continuous suture, if a single knot unties, or if the suture breaks, the entire suture line dehisces. This tends to make surgeons use heavier suture material, with a consequent increase in both tissue reaction and in the size of needle bites taken in the tissue. Many surgeons leave a continuous suture in the skin too long, and resultant scarring may be unsightly.

### Technique

The surgeon first places an ordinary single cuticular suture at one end of the incision and applies several well-squared knots. Either the needle holder or the hands may be used for this tying, but the needle holder will allow the surgeon the use of a shorter short end in tying his knots and the consequent saving of a longer portion of the suture for sewing.

The surgeon should choose the proper end of the incision to begin sewing. If the incision runs transversely from the surgeon's right to left, a right-handed surgeon should begin his running suture at the left end of the closure (Fig. 6.23A). In that way, he may conveniently supinate his right wrist in passing his needle through first the far and then the near skin margin with each bite. His left hand remains free to bring the skin margins together with his fingertips or to provide counterpressure on the skin by using a sponge, a hook, or the handle of the forceps. The dominant hand thus leads the needle as the sewing continues.

If the surgeon makes the mistake of starting at the wrong end of the incision, he will find his non-dominant wrist in a position of marked hyperextension. This difficult position is shown in Figure 6.23B and should be avoided. Note that unless the left wrist is kept hyperextended, it tends to block the surgeon's vision of the needle and needle tip. The right-to-left method of sewing (for the right-handed surgeon) also causes the surgeon to place his forearms parallel to each other and rather close together. This position of the arms tends to reduce the freedom of movement of the small muscles of the hands.

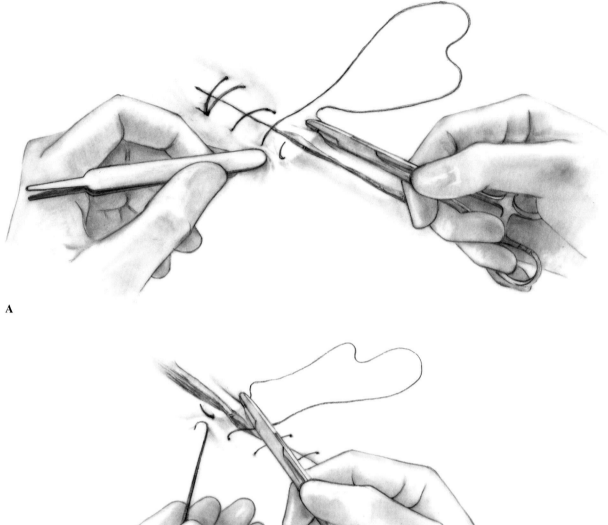

A

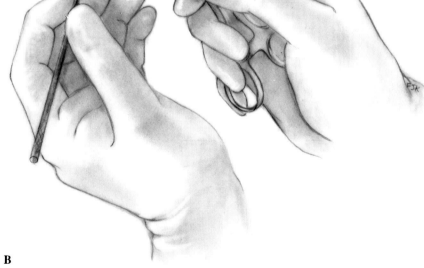

B

**Figure 6.23**

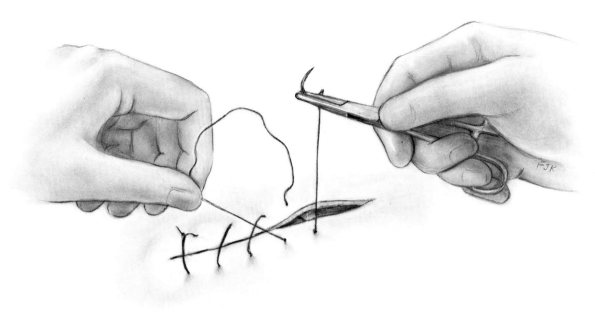

**Figure 6.24**

By the same token, a left-handed surgeon should close transverse incisions by starting at the extreme right of the wound.

When the line of closure runs at right angles to the long axis of the patient (i.e., with its long axis extending away from the surgeon toward the assistant on the opposite side of the table), the closure should always begin with the most distant part. This allows the surgeon to sew toward himself while the surgical assistant maintains modest tension on the suture and suture line without interfering with the line of vision of the surgeon as he takes the next bite with his needle (Fig. 6.24).

Continuous suture lines that approximate tissue in deep body cavities should begin at the deepest part of the suture line and progress superficially unless continuous progressive traction on more superficial tissues with each additional bite of the needle is needed to elevate and expose the margins of a deeper part of the closure.

At times the surgeon will place a continuous running suture without the aid of an assistant. He should use a method that will allow him to do this rapidly but with minimal sharp instrument handling of the skin margins. He will find it helpful to use a needle of relatively large radius and length. It may be a half-circle or a three-eighths circle in shape, but it should be long enough to reach through both sides of the skin without resetting the needle-holder. In Figure 6.25A the surgeon first everts the skin on the side of the entrance bite with the point of his skin hook, held in

his left hand. The needle holder is grasping the needle well back on its shaft. The first half of the cuticular suture is placed by pressing the needle tip straight downward. The eversion of the skin edge by the skin hook allows the needle tip to include a husky bite of the dermis (well back from the cut margin).

In Figure 6.25B the surgeon's left hand has shifted the hook to an appropriate point on the exit side of the incision. The back of the hook braces the skin margin as the needle tip first engages and then everts the wound edge. Once the skin edge is rolled outward, the needle is pushed through the skin on the second side of the incision, with the margin still held in this everted position (thus again ensuring a strong bite of deep dermis).

The counter pressure produced by the back of the skin hook assists in the delivery of the needle tip. A satisfactory alternative is for the surgeon to use the edge of his nondominant thumb or the handle end of his forceps to produce this counter pressure in lieu of the skin hook. All three methods are quite atraumatic.

Once the needle tip emerges, the hook is removed and the needle holder is then released and used (Fig. 6.25C) to grasp that portion of the needle emerg-

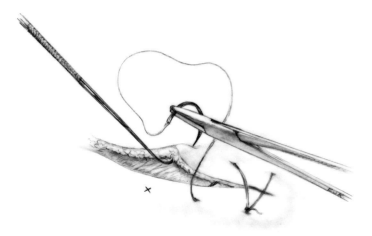

**Figure 6.25A**

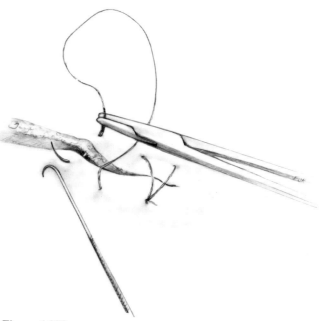

**Figure 6.25B**

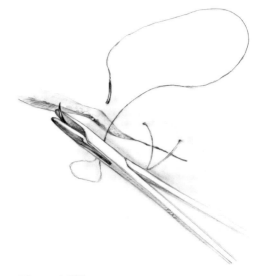

**Figure 6.25C**

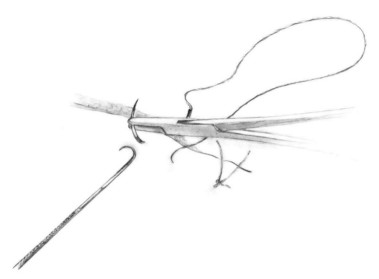

**Figure 6.25D**

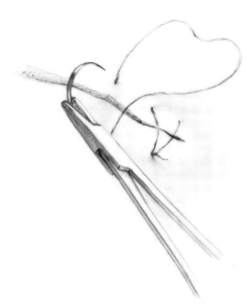

**Figure 6.25E**

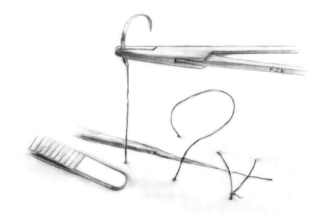

ing above the skin. In Figure 6.25*D* the needle is grasped near the tip, and the skin hook returns to again exert counterpressure during the pull. In Figure 6.25*E* the needle has been pulled almost, but not entirely, out through the skin. The butt of the needle has been deliberately left in the skin to hold the needle. The jaws of the needle holder have been loosened and

**Figure 6.25F**

allowed to slide down the curve of the needle to a point nearer the butt where the needle emerges from the skin.

In Figure 6.25*F* the needle has been clamped firmly and pulled free with a continuing further supination of the right hand and wrist. As the suture emerges, the nondominant hand first continues to offer counterforce (here with the back of a pair of forceps). This hand is then used to grasp the suture, take up the slack, and tighten the closure of the already sutured part of the incision. When there is marked tension on the closure, with wide gaping of the wound, the surgeon may have to place the bites on the near and far sides of the incision separately, thus requiring him to release and regrip the needle between each entrance and exit bite. Use of a larger needle will reduce the

need to take separate bites on the two sides of an incision during closure.

## Use of a Running Suture to Affix a Skin Graft to the Margins of a Wound

In Figure 6.26*A* a skin graft is being sutured to the margin of a wound with a running suture. In this case, the difference in thickness between the skin graft and the wound margin calls for a special method of placing the continuous suture. As the inset shows (Fig. 6.26*B*), the needle and suture pass twice through the skin graft and only once through the thicker wound margin. This ensures that some of the skin graft will cover and seal the vertical section of the wound margin. The motions of sewing are the same as shown in Figures 6.25*A–F*.

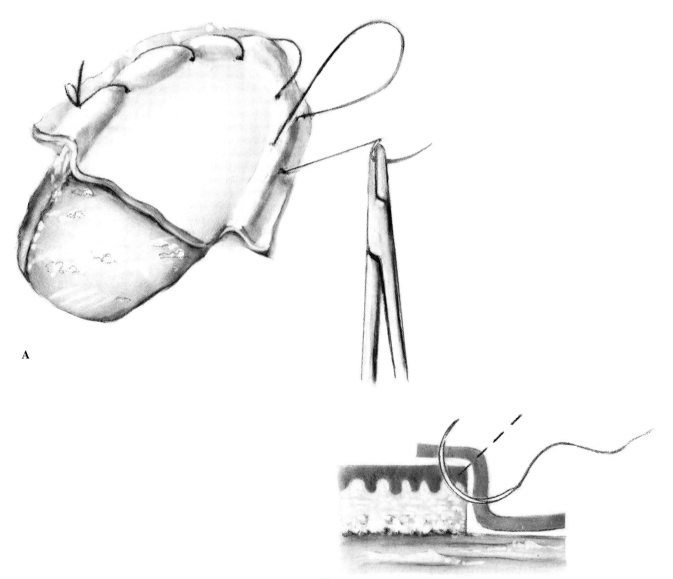

A

**Figure 6.26**          B

# Mattress Sutures

### Indications, Advantages, and Disadvantages

Interrupted or continuous mattress sutures are frequently used by general surgeons to close abdominal or chest incisions. Vertical mattress sutures are intended to gain both a secure grasp of tissue (with the large bite) and a good approximation of the skin margins (with the returning smaller bite). The concept is appealing when the skin is particularly thin and where the deep subcutaneous tissue is composed of fatty tissue that contains little firm fascia that would be suitable for the use of subcuticular sutures. There are, however, substantial drawbacks to the use of mattress sutures.

### Vertical Mattress Sutures

Figure 6.27 shows the usual method of placement of vertical mattress suture of silk or nylon. The tension required to bring the deep parts of the wound together may be greater than that which would be optimal to approximate the more superficial skin edges. Unfortunately, a mattress requires the surgeon to accept the same tension on both deep and superficial bites of the suture.

The usual crimping of skin by a mattress suture does reduce blood supply more than in the case of interrupted skin sutures. If the larger bite of the mattress suture is tight, and left in place for over 5 days, permanent wide hatchmark scars of the skin will result. These scars are difficult to correct later. They are better avoided.

*In almost every circumstance, interrupted simple cuticular sutures or a running intradermal pull-out suture will give a superior closure to that of a vertical mattress.*

### Horizontal Mattress Sutures

Horizontal mattress sutures have even less to recommend them than vertical mattress sutures. As shown in Figure 6.28, the skin that is caught within each horizontal bite will lose much of its circulation as the knot is tied. These areas of ischemia may involve up to 50% of the entire skin margin as suc-

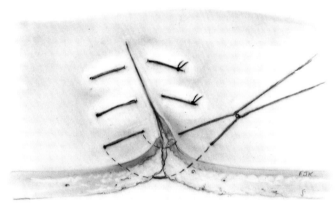

**Figure 6.27**

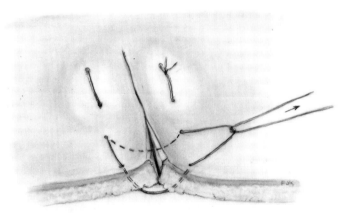

**Figure 6.28**

ceeding sutures are placed. Partial necrosis of the skin margin is not uncommon in the postoperative period when wound edema or abdominal distension adds further tension to a row of horizontal mattress sutures.

Two separate cuticular sutures will replace any horizontal mattress suture, while providing more accurate skin approximation and much-improved circulation in the intervening skin margin. There is no justification for surgeons using horizontal mattress sutures just to save a few minutes of operating time. Patients greatly appreciate meticulous skin closures in *all* parts of their bodies. It is not surprising that they assume that surgeons who leave them neat skin scars, they probably also left neat surgery beneath the skin!

## Retention or ''Stay'' Sutures

### When Indicated?

In special circumstances, the surgeon may be called on to use extremely large needles and heavy (#1 to #5) suture material. Such retention sutures are required when normal repair of deep fascia and the skin may not be expected to give secure closure. Those circumstances exist when the poor systemic condition of the patient has greatly reduced the chance for normal healing. Anemia, chronic hypoproteinemia, steroid therapy, and negative nitrogen balance may all suggest the need for retention sutures in debilitated patients.

Severe bacterial contamination of a wound or the expectation of continuing postoperative ileus and abdominal distension also increase the risk of postoperative wound dehiscence.

Advanced cancer, septic debilitation, and gross obesity are other reasons for resorting to retention sutures. They should be avoided unless one or more of these special indications are present.

### Dangers of Retention Sutures

Retention sutures to close the abdomen must be placed with great care, or the large needles that are required will injure bowel or omentum. When the sutures are tied, the loop of suture material may trap or pinch a loop of intestine. If the sutures should partially cut through the deep portion of the closed abdominal wall and allow the fascia and muscles to separate, loops of bowel may herniate upward into the deep part

of the incision. Postoperative distension may increase this process. A tight retention suture bridging a partially separated wound may cause indentation and necrosis of a bulging tense intestinal wall. Wide skin scars with crosshatch marks also frequently result from the large suture bites of retention sutures.

### Technical Precautions

The needle should be several inches in length so that it will easily penetrate the abdominal wall while the surgeon presses the abdominal viscera aside with his own nondominant hand (Fig. 6.29).

The needle is then grasped by the fingers of the surgeon or with a large needle holder and passed through the entire abdominal wall so as to include approximately half of the width of each rectus muscle and its investing fascia. With care these bites may be placed so as to include all abdominal wall tissues except the thin layer of parietal peritoneum. If this layer can be excluded from the suture bite, the danger of pinching a loop of bowel when the suture is tied will be greatly reduced. The retention sutures are left untied, but clamps are placed on each end of each retention suture as the closure proceeds. The usual layered closure of the abdominal wall fascia is then completed. The retention sutures are then tied with sufficient tension to cause slight bunching of the rectus muscles. Small segments of catheters, placed over the sutures, will cut down the tendency of these sutures to cut into the skin when postoperative distension occurs. If the abdominal wound has been grossly contaminated, a drain or loose pack may be placed in the subcutaneous space and the skin closed only loosely by tying the stay sutures. If the wound is relatively clean, cuticular sutures are placed.

Retention sutures are tied so that one or two fingers may still be slipped between the suture and the skin. Such sutures may be left in place for two or three weeks, or until clinical evidence of good abdominal wall healing is observed. The correction of any underlying anemia, hypoproteinemia or other systemic deficiency should be accomplished as rapidly as feasible.

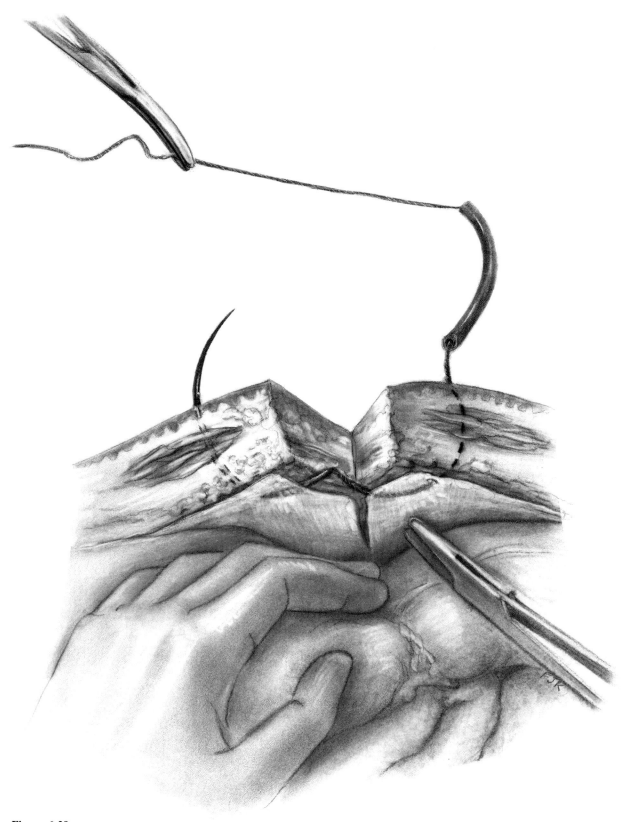

**Figure 6.29**

## Special Suturing Techniques

### Suturing in Narrow Deep Spaces

When called upon to place a suture in a very deep recess or body cavity, the surgeon may need to improvise on technique. The needle holder may need long handles, and it may be difficult to get forceps or light into the depths while sewing.

One technique of value (Fig. 6.30) may be to set the needle obliquely into the jaws of the needle holder. If one jaw of the needle holder is "windowed" (Fig. 6.30, *inset*), this may be easier. In this way, the needle may be positioned so that its point will enter the tissue almost parallel to the long axis of the needle holder. Once the needle tip has been engaged in the tissue in the correct direction, the needle holder can be released and used to push the rest of the needle through the tissue by regrasping it nearer the swage.

At times, even a small half-circle curved needle will not have enough curve to allow its tip to reappear in a narrow and limited space. Fortunately, most surgical needles are sufficiently malleable that a needle holder may be used to increase (or decrease) the curve. Figure 6.31 shows a half-circle needle, the method of bending, and the resultant needle shape that will allow it to get into (and out of) a very narrow space.

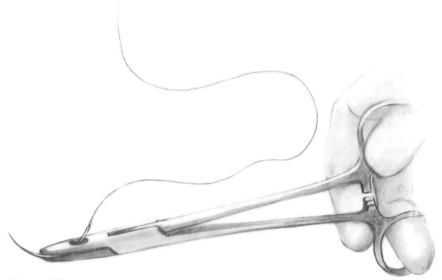

**Figure 6.30**

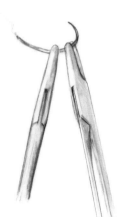
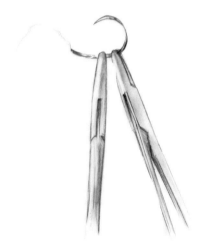

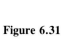
**Figure 6.31**

## Suturing With Advancement and Sewing Around Curves

When injuries or incisions produce markedly curved skin margins, problems in approximation arise as a result of the inherently different ways that normal elastic fibers in skin act on the concave and convex sides of the wound.

Figure 6.32A shows a typical pattern of skin retraction that results from a skin cut in the shape of a parabolic curve. The cut concave margin still remains close to its normal position, but the elastic fibers in the central or convex margin are now unopposed on the periphery, and the skin is consequently retracted in all dimensions.

Proper suturing of such a wound overcomes the unbalanced retraction and returns the tip of the flap to the position shown in Figure 6.32B. The method of suturing should avoid placing undue tension in the sutures used in the tip of the flap.

To precisely reposition such a flap without using high-tension tip sutures, the technique of "suturing with advancement" is used. Starting with the base of the flap and working toward the tip, interrupted cuticular sutures are placed on both sides. Each suture is placed obliquely so that, when tied, the edge of the retracted flap is advanced 1 or 2 mm further toward the tip of the defect. If a skin hook or suture is placed distally in the flap (Fig. 6.32C), it may be used to hold the flap in an advanced position as each suture is placed and tied. If proper bites of dermis are taken and skin eversion is gained, a gentle elevated ridge of skin (Halsted's roll) will be noted running along the completed suture line. The closeups in Figure 6.32D show how the sutures are placed at slightly different levels on either side of the skin, but as the flap is advanced, the suture is tied so that the loop crosses the incision line at right angles.

As one continues with this "suture with advancement" technique, the tip of the flap will begin to lie easily in its proper position (Fig. 6.32B) even before any sutures are placed in the flap tip. *This means that little tension will be needed on the final sutures used for approximation of that part of the flap which has the most precarious blood supply.*

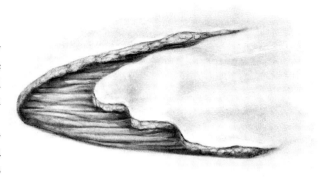

A

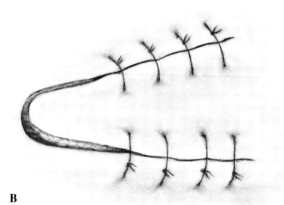

B

**Figure 6.32**

The late healing of all sharply curved skin incisions will always tend to cause a trap-door deformity, manifested by an upward bulging of skin trapped on the inside of the curve. This appearance is due to the purse-string effect of longitudinal scar contracture along the long axis of the curve. Plastic surgeons are familiar with methods to correct late trap-door deformities, but early suture with advancement is one way of minimizing this problem.

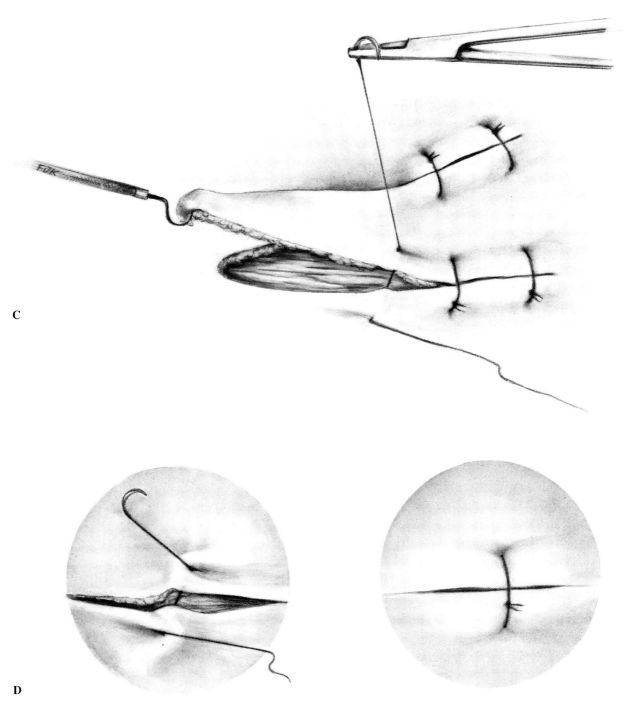

C

D

**Figure 6.32** *(continued)*

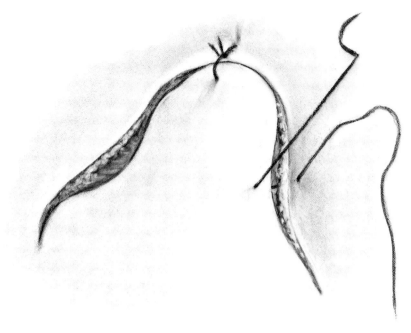

**Figure 6.33**

## Suturing by Bisection

Both straight and curved incisions may be accompanied by uneven contraction of elastic fibers on the two sides of the wound with resultant transverse shifting of one skin margin more than the other. In addition to varying pull from released elastic fiber, this uneven displacement may be increased by a greater impact of gravity on the more dependent site of the wound, by a greater adherence of the skin to the underlying fascia on one side of the wound as a result of trauma or dissection, or by the loss or removal of skin or scar on one side of the wound.

The proper alignment of skin margins of complex incisions may be greatly facilitated by placing the first cuticular (or subcuticular) suture in the exact midpoint of each side of the incision. Once this suture is tied, the remaining parts of the wound may be checked by brief manual apposition. The original trial suture may need to be replaced if it proves to be out of position. Once satisfied with its location, each of the two remaining halves of the wound are closed by further bisecting sutures that bring these secondary midpoints together.

In Figure 6.33 this principle of ''suture by bisection'' is demonstrated. Note that the first suture does much to realign the entire skin margin.

## Closure of a Skin Defect or Donor Site With Local Tissues

Frequently skin has been lost as a result of trauma, the removal of an unsightly or dangerous lesion, or the transfer of a flap or skin graft to another area of the body. In such circumstances, the donor defect may be closed by (a) simple infolding sutures without undermining, (b) undermining and margin advancement, (c) local rotation or transpositional skin flaps, or (d) skin grafting.

The closure of a simple full-thickness skin graft donor site will illustrate many of these options. The size of the defect, mobility of surrounding skin, location on the body, and thickness of the dermis in that region will all affect the surgeon's choice of method.

A

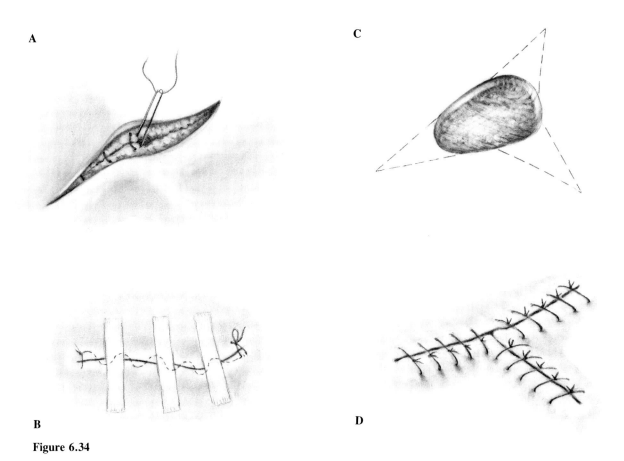

C

B

D

**Figure 6.34**

Figure 6.34*A* and *B* show an excellent method of closure when an elliptical graft of moderate size has been removed from a mobile area such as the groin. In Figure 6.34*A* the residual deep dermis is being rolled or infolded on itself by subcuticular interrupted sutures of fine nylon. The skin edges are not undermined, but they are brought closer together as the dermis is plicated. With thin skin, the nylon should be placed several millimeters away from the skin margins. The knots are placed on the deep side of the loop. The second and third layers of closure are shown in Figure 6.34*B*. A running buried intradermal prolene suture has been placed after tying it above the skin surface at one end. Steri-strips (skin adhesive tapes) have been added to improve epidermal approximation in three areas and to reduce postoperative tension and movement of the skin margins.

In Figure 6.34*C* a more circular type of defect in some donor areas may lend itself to a different pattern of closure. By the removal of three small triangles as shown in the dotted areas, the defect is converted into a shape that can be closed in a T or a Y shape. After a few subcuticular sutures are placed, interrupted silk cuticular sutures complete the closure. This method should only be used when there is minimal slackness of the skin in both the vertical and horizontal directions and when there is no clearly dominant line of skin relaxation. Angular or T-shaped closures, as shown in Figure 6.34*D*, are usually approximated more accurately by interrupted sutures than by the running intradermal technique. Even so, these three-limbed scars usually heal less satisfactory than a straight or slightly curved closure.

## Proper Tension on Sutures

### History

Sutures that are too tight cut into the skin and deep tissue. This tightness cuts off blood supply, scars the skin, causes postoperative pain and discomfort, and delays healing. If sutures are very tight, ischemic gangrene of some part of the wound may result.

Sutures that are too loose fail to approximate skin and deeper tissues and allow continuous motion between the wound interfaces. This motion breaks down bridging and early healing, stimulates excessive collagen synthesis, delays the sealing off of the wound, and encourages the collection of blood and serum in the dead spaces.

How does the surgeon manage to keep the tension of his sutures between this Scylla and this Charybdis?

In the early 19th century, Von Graefe and other German surgeons utilized small carved sticks of orange wood to regulate suture tension. The ends of each suture were passed through an eye in a stick and then wound about a fish-tailed split in its opposite end (Fig. 6.35). Each day the surgeon would loosen or tighten the suture as the postoperative wound edema came and went. These early surgeons certainly appreciated that attention to such detail paid off handsomely in surgical healing! Modern surgeons have less tedious methods of securing proper suture tension.

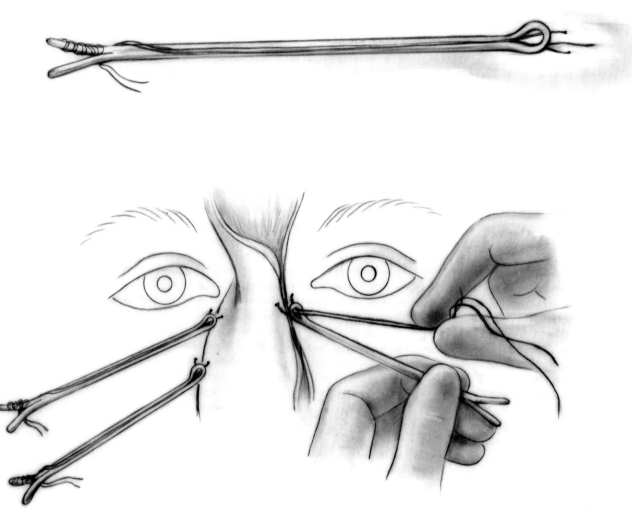

**Figure 6.35**

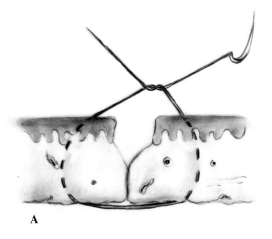

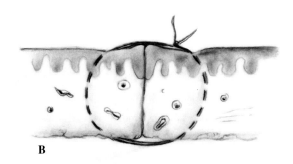

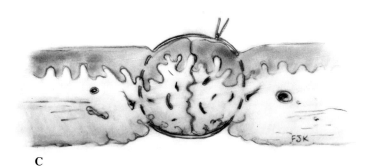

**Figure 6.36**

## Judging Tension

When a skin suture is tied, it first draws the margins of the wound together. If the bite has been properly placed (Fig. 6.36*A*), the deep portions of the wound should be brought together before the skin margins. As the suture is tightened further, the tissue gathered within the bite of the suture is compressed into a more circular cross-section (Fig. 6.36*B*). The skin edges first make contact approximation, and then the skin at the site of the closed incision rises slightly above the surrounding skin surface. This is the proper tension. The knot should then be squared and set.

If the tension is increased above the optimal level, the skin margins will tend to overlap or become inverted, the capillaries in the dermis become compressed (Fig. 6.36*C*), and the external surface of the skin will show a faint pallor around the exit points of the suture. Tension will increase even further after an additional 24 to 48 hours as a result of postoperative interstitial edema. Even if the circulation of the skin survives such a tight suture, the skin will be ''cut'' and permanently scarred within a few days, and wound tensile strength, at the time of normal suture removal on the fifth postoperative day, may be reduced by 50% to 75% (in comparison to a wound sutured under ideal tension).

If the young surgeon will take the trouble to test this effect by deliberately setting his sutures too tightly over one-half of the length of a few of his suture lines, he may compare subsequent healing and scar formation of this half of the incision with the other half (where suture tension produced gentle but snug closure). He will quickly get convincing evidence of the drawbacks of tight sutures and improve his skills in judging proper suture tension. Even experienced surgeons have a tendency to tie sutures too tightly. It seems to be a problem of human nature.

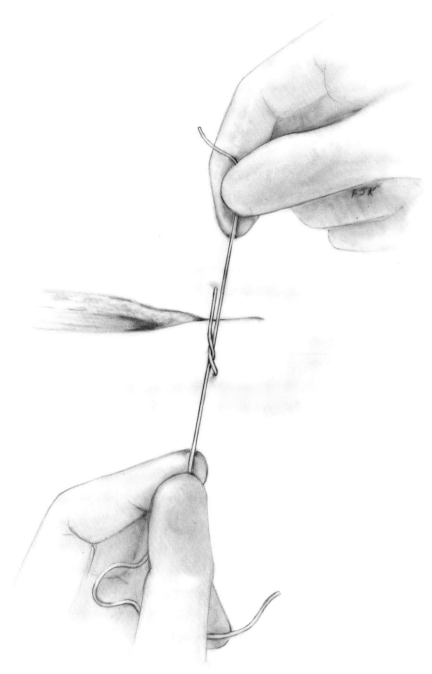

**Figure 6.37A**

## Setting Proper Knot Tension

Once he has learned to estimate the desired tightness of skin closure, the surgeon must have rapid and dependable methods of setting the first throw of his knots so that the tension remains at that optimum level. The ease of setting knot tension depends on both materials and technique.

## Silk

Silk continues to have the best ''hand'' qualities of all suture materials. The surgeon can set his first knot with less danger of it slipping than with any other flexible suture material. Usually, he may draw the skin together with a single-loop laid flat. If there is tension on the closure he may elect to ''set'' the loop of his first throw by holding the long near end of the

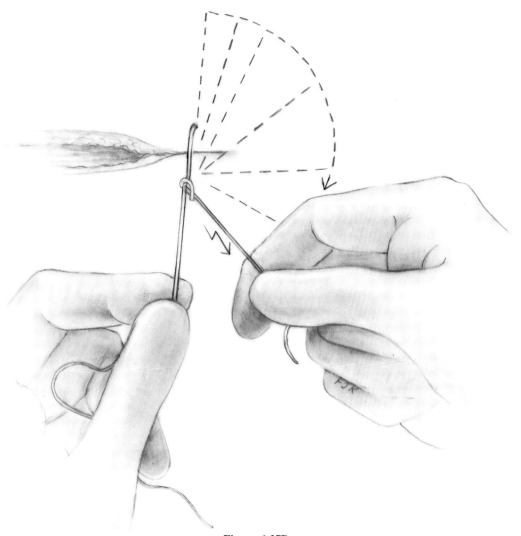

**Figure 6.37B**

suture taut as he swings the short end back through a 180° arc and gives it a light jerk at the end of the arc so as to double the suture beneath itself. This sets the first throw, and it is held by the tension on the loop (Fig. 6.37A–B). The pull on the two held ends of the "locked" suture is then relaxed, and kept relaxed, until a second throw has been added that will square the knot. This may be done with a two-handed tie (Figs. 5.8 and 5.9) or by means of a tie technique using a needle holder. Some skill is needed to draw this second loop down completely and firmly before *exerting any tension* on either suture end. Premature tension on either end of the suture will loosen the first loop and require that it be reset. Additional knots are

added for security. Tying by this method also allows the surgeon to place the knot well to one side of the suture line. This lateral location of the knot reduces the postoperative collection of crusts in the knots and improves skin edge approximation. It also assists with proper elevation of the dermis along the suture line as the knot is tightened.

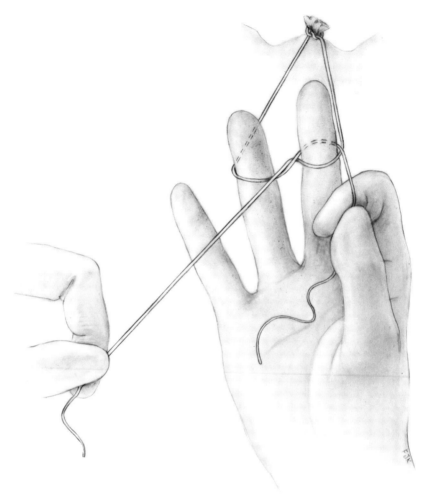

**Figure 6.38**

Some degree of tension on the wound closure is actually helpful in keeping the set loop in position after locking. However, if the incision requires marked tension for closure, even silk may slip after a single loop is locked. In these cases, an initial double loop or ''surgeon's knot'' is placed. This will usually hold, even when laid flat, if there is significant tension on the closure. Again, as in Figure 6.38 and 6.44, the second knot should be tied while keeping both ends of the suture without tension so as not to jiggle loose the first loop until the second has been firmly set. Either the one-handed or two-handed method may be effective for tying a knot without placing tension on either suture end. A one-handed knot (Fig. 6.38) may be tied in the same fashion with either hand.

Very occasionally, closures must be done under great tension. When this is so, the assistant should use skin hooks or other retractors to draw such wound margins together as each suture is being tied. Even a surgeon's knot may tend to slip as a result of the tension. Here the surgeon must use a technique of tying under tension. The first knot is set, and both ends are held taut as a one-handed method of tying is used to place the second loop (Fig. 6.39). Alternatively, a two-handed method of placing the second loop may be used (as shown in Figs. 5.8 and 5.9). Again, this second loop is pulled down without releasing the tension on either end of the suture. This method will sometimes result in sawing and runs some risk of breaking of the suture material. The surgeon's glove, especially if thin or loose-fitting, may get caught in the suture as the loop is formed and pulled tightly over the surgeon's fingertip. A bit of practice is needed to smoothly tie under tension and avoid catching the glove.

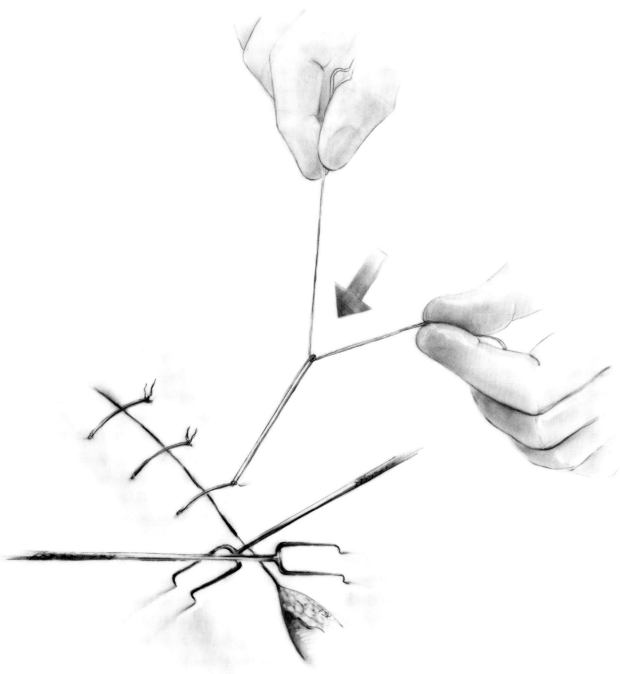

**Figure 6.39**

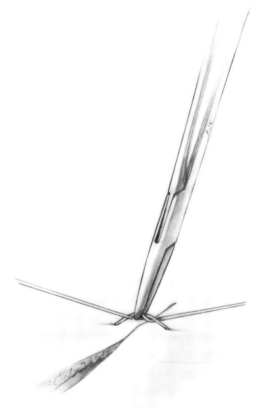

**Figure 6.40**

matter of luck when it produces the proper amount of tension on the suture.

When very small sutures and small bites of skin are used, one should avoid the use of a surgeon's knot. Any double first loop, when laid flat, is rather wide and will often extend across both skin margins and cause a crimping of the skin and irregular approximation (Fig. 6.41A). One advantage of using silk when small skin bites are needed is that it seldom requires a surgeon's knot on the first throw to set proper knot tension (Fig. 6.41B).

### Absorbable sutures

Absorbable suture materials such as catgut, dexon, or vicryl have easily roughened surfaces. They tend to fray as they are tied under tension. They are most often used as buried sutures and are placed well beneath the skin. They are useful where closure or positioning of deep tissue by suture is only required for a few days or weeks after surgery.

Rarely, the surgeon will be tying with such heavy suture material and under such tension that he will ask his assistant to pinch the first loop of his knot with a smooth-jawed needle holder until he can form and set the second knot. When this method is used, the assistant must be careful to grasp the knot with only the very tip of the needle holder (Fig. 6.40) and to release it without sawing the suture material with the edge of the needle holder. To do so will break or weaken the suture.

### Synthetic suture materials

Nylon and prolene suture loops have low coefficients of friction and will slide more easily than silk, but they do not set as securely and they require a larger number of knots on each suture to avoid later loosening of the knot. If there is significant wound tension on closure, these materials (unlike silk) will *routinely* require that a surgeon's (double loop) knot be used as the first throw.

The practice of loosely tying a "granny knot" and then trying to tighten this double loop to the proper degree should be discouraged. Accurate control of the tightening is impossible and, it is largely a

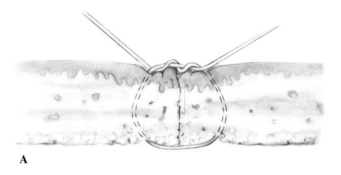

A

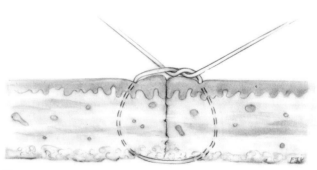

B

**Figure 6.41**

Absorbable sutures do play a useful role in skin suturing in children, in whom suture removal may be painful or difficult, and on parts of the body where skin scarring from suture marks is not of high importance. An example would be the use of catgut sutures to close the skin of the hand in children under the age of 6 or 8 years.

Sutures about the vagina, perineum, genitalia, and within the oral cavity are most often appropriately of absorbable suture material since suture mark scars are of minimal importance in those areas.

### Metallic sutures

Steel wire may be used for skin closure. The finest gauge required should be used. The alloy should be one that allows bending and pulling without breaking. A stiff or brittle wire conforms poorly to the tissues being approximated.

Wire may be tied with a two-handed tie or with a needle holder. The first loop must be formed flat and kept flat by drawing it down while keeping both ends of the wire well apart (Fig. 6.42A). The second loop must also be constructed without exerting tension on either end of the wire, and this flat loop is drawn down to square the knot. Each end of the wire is then lifted slightly and separately cut off close to the knot (Fig. 6.42B). If the two ends of the wire are brought together, held up, and cut with a single motion of the scissors, the second knot will lose its flat form, become looped, and usually come untied. Steel wire is very nonreactive and can be effective as a suture material, but different and special techniques are needed to handle it with efficiency.

# Role of the Surgical Assistant in Suturing

Suturing in most operations will occur largely at the time of wound closure. In some surgical specialties, such as plastic surgery, suturing may be a conspicuous part of the procedure early in the surgery, or even at several different times during an operation.

The surgical assistant can do much to expedite suturing. If the scrub nurse is relatively new to the procedure, and if she has not checked with the surgeon to find out what needles and sutures he will want for closing, the assistant should raise the question himself unless he already knows that surgeon's preference.

As closure time approaches, the assistant should check the field to be sure that all packs and sponges are recovered from wound recesses. Any remaining bleeders in the angles of the wound should be identified and controlled. Moist sponges may be used to cover any exposed surfaces that appear dry, and others may be used to clean clots from the skin around the wound margins. Overhead lights may need adjustment to improve illumination of the field, retractors may need repositioning for better visibility, and equipment for final wound irrigation may be readied for use.

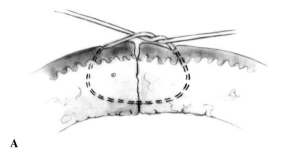

A

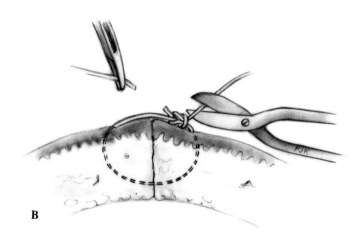

B

**Figure 6.42**

All of these support activities should be completed quietly, while keepng one eye on the surgeon and remaining alert to help him with more specific activities. At times, the surgeon will assign to the assistant a specific task such as stopping a bleeder, inserting a drain, or closing a part of the wound or donor site. In the absence of such an assignment, the assistant should direct his efforts toward a smooth flow of motion in the primary operative field. He must take care, for example, not to put his hand or arm in the surgeon's line of vision (Fig. 6.43) as he obtains instruments or returns them to the scrub nurse. Thus, passage of arms and instruments will always occur outside of the "visual cones" that extend from the eyes of the surgical team to the operative field. These exchanges can be made beneath the surgeon's arms and along the sides of the table without interrupting the operation (Fig. 6.43). The assistant should never reach behind the surgeon's back to get an instrument, and his hands should always remain above elbow level if he is to avoid risk of touching an unsterile surface.

## Who Will Tie the Knots?
## Who Will Cut the Sutures?

Once a surgeon has worked with a given assistant for several weeks, he may prefer to have the assistant tie his knots while he obtains the next suture and needle and prepares for the next stitch. This is an efficient system, but only if the assistant has developed a reliable skill with tying. The assistant must find a smooth and graceful way to take the needle and its suture. He must tie the first knot with the proper tension and without breaking the suture. He should be able to lock sutures on the first try when tying under tension, then be able to rapidly, and automatically, throw on several additional squared knots. He must efficiently present both ends of the suture to the surgeon (or second assistant) in proper position for cutting, and quickly return the needle and remaining suture material to the scrub nurse. All of this should be done *before* the surgeon has placed the first bite of the next suture in the tissues.

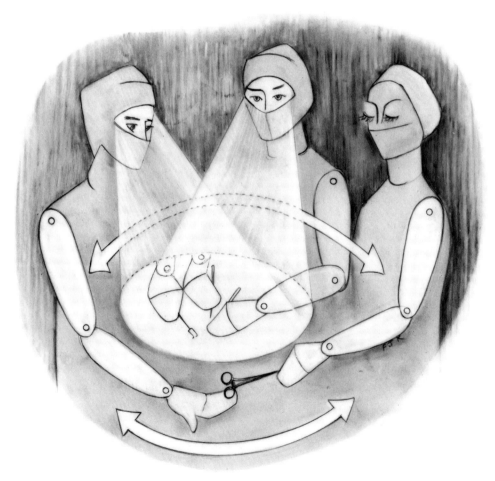

**Figure 6.43**

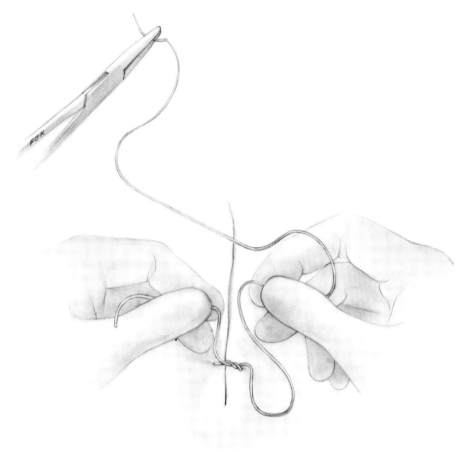

**Figure 6.44**

If the assistant uses a slow or unreliable method of tying, if he breaks many sutures by rough pulls, or if he tightens the first knots excessively, he should not be surprised to find the surgeon beginning to tie his own knots as he sutures.

One of the secrets of doing surgery rapidly is to avoid having to repeat numerous operative steps. If a bleeder requires repeated ties or coagulations to control it, if a suture has to be loosened or replaced in a new location, or if retractors are not positioned well on the first attempt, the operation will be slowed and extra trauma will be inflicted on the tissues.

The assistant may wish to check with the surgeon to find out whether he would like to recover his own needles as the suturing begins. If several stitches are to be taken with each swaged on needle and suture, the surgeon will usually withdraw the needle from the tissue with his own needle holder. The assistant may

then pull the remaining extra length of suture through the tissue, leaving only enough length on the short end to allow him to tie rapidly and accurately. When tying for the surgeon, the assistant will have already grasped the short end of the suture as the surgeon was starting to place this stitch, in anticipation of this knotting. He should use a two-handed tie that allows him to tie and square this knot without causing the surgeon to relinquish his hold on the needle (Fig. 6.44). While the knot is being tied, the surgeon will usually reposition the needle in his needle holder for the next bite and be sure that the suture scissors are readied for cutting the suture. Once the suture is cut, the assistant discards the short end, but retains a grip on the long end if the surgeon continues to use this same needle and suture to place the next bite. This process continues until the suture becomes too short for convenient tying. At that point, the scrub nurse provides another.

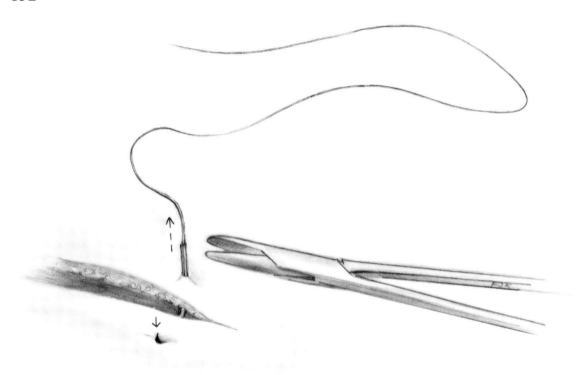

**Figure 6.45A**

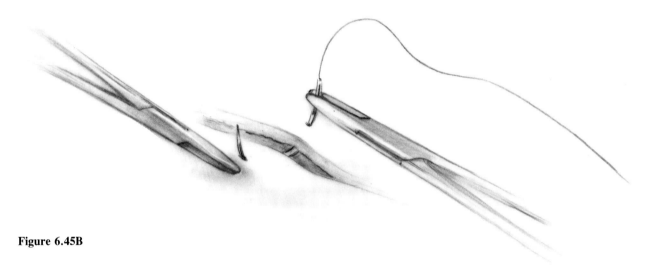

**Figure 6.45B**

### Needle Fixation and Presentation

Sometimes the tension on the closure, the thickness of the tissues, or the relatively small size of the needle may make it difficult for the surgeon to grasp the emerging tip of his needle. If, at that point, he releases the needle holder, the wound tension may pull the needle back below the surface (Fig. 6.45A). If his nondominant hand is engaged in bringing the wound edges together, he may need a third hand to grasp the needle tip as it comes into view. When this is the situation, the assistant should quickly make the diagnosis and be ready with a needle holder. He should first use the closed tip of the needle holder to provide counterforce downward alongside the point of the needle to aid its penetration (Fig. 6.45B). Then, when the surgeon pauses after completing his ''supinating push,'' of the needle holder, the assistant grasps the needle firmly just behind the point, taking care not to bend or blunt it (Fig. 6.45C). The surgeon then unlocks his needle holder, and the assistant rotates the needle 90° through its natural curve. This brings most

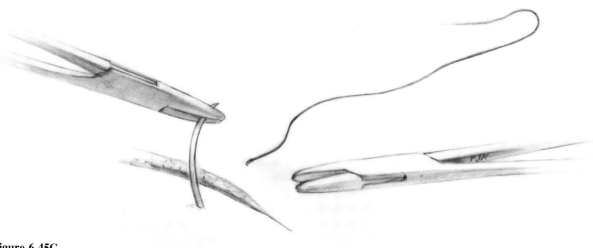

**Figure 6.45C**

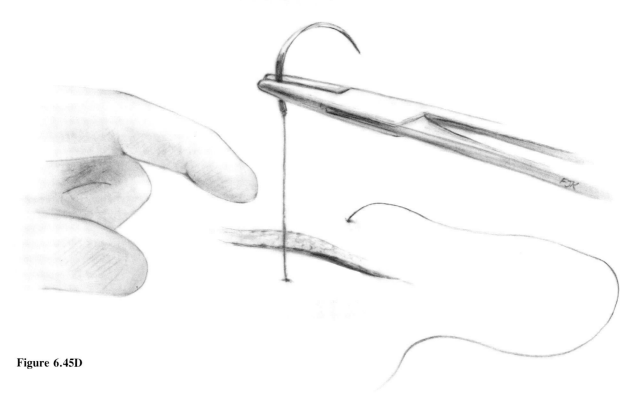

**Figure 6.45D**

of the needle above the skin surface, but *care is taken to leave the butt of the needle still beneath the skin.* The fixation of the needle between the skin below and the assistant's needle holder above makes it stable and easy for the surgeon to grasp. He does so and then completes the removal of the needle from the tissue as the assistant reaches for the suture when it emerges behind the needle (Fig. 6.45*D*) and then begins the first throw of his knot. This technique is known as "needle fixation and presentation," and it may be of much value in deep cavity suturing, as well as in wound closure.

## Anticipating Needs for Drains and Dressings

As wound closure proceeds, the assistant should anticipate the possible need for drains, suction, and dressings. If he has not worked with the surgeon for very long, he should raise the question and ask the nurse to secure the proper size and type of equipment. He may be able to place a drain and suture it in position without slowing the surgeon's rhythm of wound closure.

Dressings have many functions (see Chapter 7), but the scrub nurse should have all packaged materials opened and the needed items ready before the drapes are removed. She should check, before passing off her instruments or leaving the operating table until the dressings have been completed. Dressings are critical parts of many operations and premature abandonment of the surgical field by the scrub nurse is one of the commonest errors in modern operating room routines.

### Discussing Postoperative Management and Dangers

As the routine of wound closure is established, the surgical assistant should review plans for postoperative care with the surgeon. The latter, if experienced, will usually know what the greatest risks will be for that operation. Orders to prevent, anticipate, detect, and correct such problems can be discussed. Special postoperative routines and information that should be given to relatives are reviewed. A final check with the anesthesiologist will coordinate surgical postoperative needs of the patient.

### Educational Activities During the Operation

The surgical assistant who has fulfilled his responsibilities as an alert, intelligent, informed, and skilled facilitator has a right to expect the experience in the operating room to add to his personal education. *It is rare to find an outstanding surgeon who was not once an outstanding assistant!*

In every operation, there comes a time when the critical decisions have been made and the most demanding technical challenges have been met. The sewing and tying may not be complete, but the die is cast. The success or failure of the surgery will have largely been determined. At that point, the assistant should feel free to show the depth of his interest in the operation. He may inquire about alternative procedures the surgeon might have used. He may wish to discuss the pathology, prognosis, or management of possible postoperative complications.

The surgeon will usually welcome such genuine interest on the part of the assistant and will usually answer such questions as best he can. In turn, he may choose to question the assistants in order to assess the level of sophistication they have reached and perhaps to imply what sorts of things they should already have learned at their various levels of training.

All of this should be in a serious but good-natured vein. *Surgeons should enjoy their work!* Any job that offers variety and surprise, while providing relief of disease and deformity to fellow humans, should be highly gratifying. Badly done surgery is seldom rewarding to anyone.

# 7

## Dressings, Drains, and Suture Removal

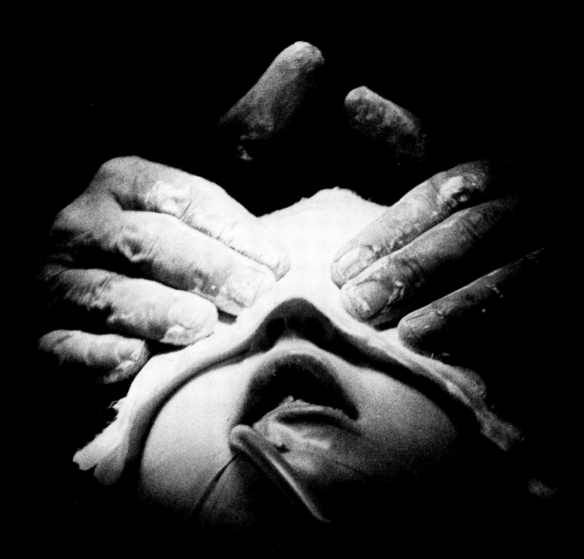

# 7

## Dressings, Drains, and Suture Removal

# Dressings—Art or Skill?

Bradford Cannon once told the author that he could always tell a knowledgeable visiting surgeon from an unsophisticated one, because the former always stayed in the operating room to watch how the dressing was applied, while the latter went out to get a cup of coffee as he waited for the start of the next case.

The immediate postoperative management of surgical wounds has the potential for either aiding or damaging the healing process. A thoughtless or improperly applied dressing may completely destroy or undo the painstaking work in the operating room that preceded it.

Good surgical dressings require both art and skill. The surgeon must use the proper materials and, above all, must develop the knowledge of how to apply them and when to apply them. He depends on the sense of touch in his fingers to secure them under the proper tension. His goals are to secure wound support and protection, while leaving the patient comfortable. The latter should not have the uneasy sensation that the dressing might loosen or come off unexpectedly during the postoperative period. Unfortunately, the art and skills of applying surgical dressings are in danger of being lost. These techniques are seldom well demonstrated to young surgical residents.

Hairy areas of skin should be shaved before applying adhesive tape. Skin should be protected with a solution such as compound tincture of benzoin or mastisol. These solutions will also improve dressing security by increasing tape adhesiveness. Tape should support (reduce) skin tension on the closure, but not be applied so tightly as to cause shear blistering.

Wrapped dressings should be molded and contoured to the body parts so as to avoid postoperative shifting. Opposing skin surfaces should be separated by gauze and powder before wrapping. Ears should not be wrapped tightly against the head, and fingers should not be compressed tightly together over a wedge of padding in the depth of their common web. To do so may occlude circulation through the digital vessels.

The surgeon will do well to remember that the patient will view his dressing (regardless of who applied it) and inevitably make judgments from it about the skill and carefulness of the surgery that preceded it.

# Purposes of Dressings and Drains

## Wound Protection

A dressing should be used only when it has a clear and definite function. Some dressings are only protective. They are used to avoid external trauma or to keep the patient's fingers from doing harm to the wound. A simple absorbent gauze pad, well fixed with tape around the wound margins, will often suffice. If there is any area of open wound, the gauze that contacts the wound surface should be of fine mesh (#30 gauze) to avoid penetration of it by the subsequent ingrowth of buds of granulation tissue. Ingrowth of budding capillaries will cause pain on removal of

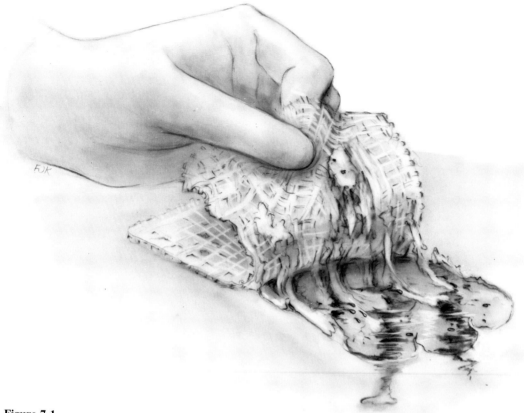

**Figure 7.1**

dressings. Figure 7.1 shows how the removal of a coarse mesh dry gauze dressing from a granulating wound, after several days of application, will cause renewed bleeding as the blood vessels that have grown into the gauze are torn. The thin and delicate new epithelium that has formed along the wound margins is also stripped away. The removal of such a dressing may be quite painful. All of this could have been avoided if fine mesh xeroform[1] gauze had been used to dress the wound.

In dressing hand wounds on children, it is prudent to use elbow splints. These are often applied in the recovery room. They prevent elbow flexion and keep the child from reaching the wound with his fingers, while leaving the arms free for motion at the shoulder joints.

### Promotion of Wound Drainage

Wounds or incisions that are infected or significantly contaminated with bacteria will heal more promptly if drainage is promoted sufficiently to ensure that fluids are not trapped within the wound. This may

[1]Xeroform ointment has the advantage of having a beeswax base that causes less skin maceration than petrolatum.

be accomplished by the use of moist or wet dressings. The moisture prevents the scab and crust formation that occurs with drying on exposure to air. Liquid exudates are thus not blocked and will continue to escape into the dressing in the days that follow surgery. The normal mechanisms of wound healing are aided by allowing this removal of detritus and necrotic material. Desiccation of a wound surface delays healing.

Another method of promoting drainage is the use of ointment or ointment-impregnated gauze on the surface of suture lines or open wounds. This also retards drying and crust formation and reduces the adherence of gauze. The removal of ointment-impregnated gauze is less painful than dry gauze when dressings are changed.

Many ointments have a vaseline or petrolatum base. At times their oil molecules may become trapped in the healing wound and produce a troublesome "paraffinoma." For this reason, many surgeons prefer to use an ointment that contains a beeswax base. Beeswax is much less likely to be captured within the healing tissue. Some excellent water-soluble ointment bases are also available and quite useful in gauze impregnation.

Once sufficient sutures have been placed around the margin of a skin graft, a large square of greasy fine mesh gauze is laid over the wound. Dry cotton or well-fluffed gauze is placed over the greased gauze, the edges of which are folded up over the cotton and compressed by the fingers of the surgical assistant as the sutures are tied. The amount of cotton in the bolus should be sufficient to create a sphere, when compressed, of a large enough diameter that the sutures will be required to diverge outward from the margin of the graft before they can converge over the top of the bolus (Fig. 7.3B). If the bolus is too small, good graft-to-bed apposition will not be obtained along the margins of the defect.

The surgeon will usually tie the sutures in pairs, selecting for each knot two adjacent sutures from opposite sides of the graft. He ties a single loop and draws it down firmly. As he does so, the assistant firms up the bolus with the fingers of one hand and presses the cotton down firmly with the tip of a closed smooth-jawed needle holder. When the surgeon pauses, having tightened the knot to proper tension, the assistant uses the jaw tips of his needle holder to fix the knot (Fig. 7.4). The surgeon then adds a second throw. If the greased gauze catches in the knot, it is wise for the assistant also to fix the second throw with his needle holder. Four or five additional throws are then added. Two more pairs of suture ends are selected and tied in similar fashion.

This process continues until the sutures are all secured. Additional grease impregnated gauze is then draped over the bolus and snugged into the angle between the skin and the base of the bolus (to prevent sticking at the time of first dressing). The outer dressing is then built up around the bolus with more cotton. The entire dressing is wrapped or taped so as to prevent its dislodgement by accidental blows or pressure. Attention to such details in applying a bolus dressing will pay off in highly reliable results and consistent 100% graft takes.

The completed dressing (shown in Fig. 7.3B) was secured by leaving only one end of each silk suture long after tying. These single long ends were then all tied over the bolus. However, when prolonged immobilization of the graft is required, as in grafting a child below the age of cooperation, both ends of each suture used in the graft margin may be left long. One end of each suture may be used to tie over the initial bolus, while the second "reserve" set of long ends are simply folded and laid on the surface of the graft before being covered by the gauze and cotton. When the first set of suture ends are clipped on the sixth day after surgery, the bolus is removed, the graft checked, any blood or serum is released, and the loose second end of each suture used to tie on a second bolus of cotton for an additional week of secure fixation.

In most situations a tie-on bolus is needed for only one postoperative week, and all sutures usually are removed at the time of that first dressing.

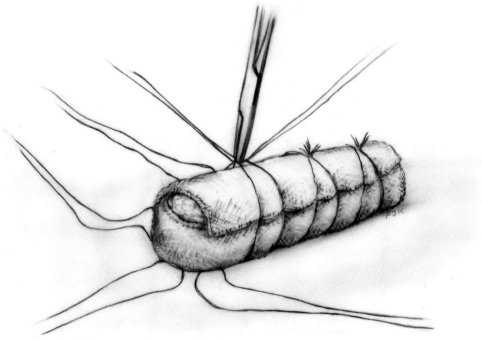

**Figure 7.4**

## Plaster of Paris casts and other rigid external dressings

Plaster of Paris splints and rigid synthetic casts are but another form of dressing used to hold an injured part in stable position until healing is complete. Rigid external dressings create a type of temporary exoskeleton to replace the strength of tissue support lost when the human internal skeleton is broken. Members of the insect world of course normally depend on a biological exoskeleton for their tissue support. In a sense, they wear a "natural" cast to protect their internal tissues.

Casts have great value in substituting for bone and in allowing fractures to heal, but they also are of considerable use as dressings for soft tissue injury and repair. They may be used to hold joints or fingers in flexed or extended positions so as to prevent undue tension on a repaired nerve or tendon.

In Figure 7.5 a cast has been used to splint the elbow, wrist, and fingers in modest flexion following the repair of the profundus long flexor tendon to the ring finger. Although the elbow is not injured, the cast has been allowed to extend above the flexed elbow to prevent any tendency of the cast to shift distally. Such shifting of the cast toward the fingers would cause undesirable extending of the wrist and result in increased tension on the repaired flexor tendon. This precaution is of special importance when the patient is an active young child.

The cast is shaped closely about the wrist, and a strong flange has been extended out to the level of the proximal interphalangeal joints. This flange prevents unwanted full extension of the metacarpophalangeal joints (which might rupture the tendon repair), while at the same time it allows flexion of the metacarpophalangeal and both flexion and extension of the interphalangeal joints. This guarded mobility prevents joint stiffness from developing.

Note that all the fingertips are exposed to monitor circulation and that the cast has been trimmed back around the base of the thumb. This frees the thumb for useful motion and further avoids joint ankylosis. A metal loop has been added to the cast, and a rubber band runs from this loop to a silk suture placed in the free edge of the nail of the long finger (containing the repaired flexor tendon). This elastic band produces dynamic resistance for the uninjured long extensor tendon to work against while, at the same time, it takes tension off the freshly repaired flexor tendon.

Attention to such details in using any cast adds to the art of doing a surgical dressing.

In many cases the part of the body requiring splinting is bony and lies beneath the skin and investing muscles. Yet the principles of dressing are the same. The cast should be well padded yet fit the contours of the body surface closely enough to prevent

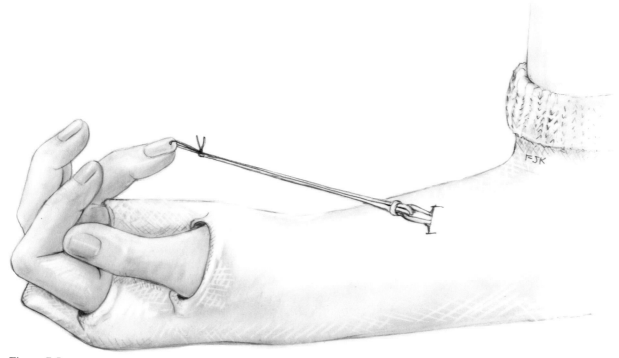

**Figure 7.5**

rubbing. It should not be so tight as to cut off circulation. Swelling and edema that may appear after cast application must be anticipated. When they are expected, the circulation should be checked at early periods (6 to 24 hours) after applying the cast. Joints that do not require splinting should be left free. Above all, a cast must fix the parts well enough to prevent motion between the bone ends at the fracture site.

A plaster cast is a special type of dressing used to supplement the normal internal fixation of tissues. The wrapping, rubbing, and smoothing of plaster as it is applied will give the cast greater strength and a more professional fit. These are skills best learned by practice. A light, strong, neat, comfortable cast is a joy for the patient and a testimonial to one of the arts of surgical dressing.

At times the use of external pin fixation, with the pins penetrating the skin and fixed in bone, may replace the use of a rigid cast. The risk of introducing infection through the skin openings and along the pin sites is present with all forms of external skeletal fixation. Good hygiene and the daily use of topical antibiotic ointment about the pin entrance sites will reduce this risk.

### Splinting of one structure to protect another

A dressing may also be used to position one part of the body so as to use that part to protect or splint another. A good example of this principle is the use of a dressing to fix the upper eyelid in a closed position so as to protect the cornea from drying or injury in the postoperative period.

Another use of this dressing principle is seen in treatment of a fracture of the upper jaw. In such patients, the teeth in the nonfractured lower jaw are wired (''dressed'') against those on both sides of the fracture in the upper. This intermaxillary fixation fixes the fractured bones and locks the teeth into the proper position of occlusion during healing. Intermaxillary fixation may also be achieved by an external wrapping such as a Barton dressing. Proper application of this dressing holds the lower jaw firmly against the upper and does not constrict the upper airway. The wrapping goes from vertex to occiput to chin, and then repeats in that order until the jaw is secure.

Teeth are thus very convenient handles on bones that assist in holding fractured jaws together. If bones in other parts of the body happened to possess teeth that projected through the skin, orthopedic surgeons would use very different ways of dressing and splinting those bones when they were fractured.

### Splinting of painful joints or muscles

When muscles or joints are inflamed as a result of infection, injury, or surgical trauma, immobilization by dressings may reduce discomfort and accelerate healing. Such dressings should place the injured body part in a functional or balanced position that will leave tendons at normal tensions and avoid malpositions that may cause secondary contractures. Footdrop may occur if a dressing or cast fails to hold the ankle in a position of modest dorsal extension. The proper dressing to prevent this complication may require only a simple splint to hold the ankle at a 90° angle, or an encircling external cast may be used.

### Dressings that elevate a body part

At times the principal function of a dressing is the simple elevation of a part of the body above the level of the heart. The part may be a lymphedematous foot or leg, or a crushed hand suffering from a reduced overflow of venous and lymphatic fluids. Overhead suspension of the injured part to the bedframe is an effective method of elevation in bedridden patients. The suspended part may be balanced with a weight and pulley so as to allow easy movement and more comfort. Alternatively, a large pillow may be pinned around the outside of a dressed extremity with large blanket pins. The thickness of the pillow elevates the extremity without the need to anchor it to a stationary bedside IV pole. This pillow technique gives the patient freedom to turn and move the limb from one side of the bed to the other. This shifting reduces shoulder joint discomfort and stiffness.

Slings or splints to support the arm also may be incorporated into the dressings of ambulatory patients to maintain elevation of the hand.

The combinations and varieties of dressings that provide elevation are limited only by the imagination of the surgeon.

### Dressings That Reduce Tissue Tension on Healing Wounds

Tension on healing wounds may be prevented in some instances by splinting to limit movements of adjacent joints (Fig. 7.5). At other times, the natural elasticity in skin or the tone and contractions of muscles on either side of a wound may work against the healing process. If not counteracted, these forces may delay healing, spread scars, or even produce a wound separation or dehiscence.

Some external dressings are helpful in preventing such tensions and thus reduce the danger of damage to the healing process.

### Adhesive skin tapes

Perhaps the most commonly used antitension dressing technique is the adhesive skin tape. These commercial tapes may be porous or impermeable, rigid or elastic.

Porous tapes allow blood and serum to drain through their perforations. These pores are shown in the tapes used in Figure 7.6A to relieve tension on a suture line. The porosity is most helpful directly over the incision itself, but some drainage will also occur from the skin that is covered by the tape on either side of the healing incision.

In this instance, the tapes are being used to supplement a row of interrupted cuticular sutures. These sutures are placed so as to help prevent the undesirable tendency of skin tapes to invert the skin margins, as illustrated in Figure 7.6B. When skin tapes alone are used to close skin incisions, there is a consistent tendency for the epidermis on either side of the incision to be rolled inward by the overlying tape. The inversion of the wound margin is particularly prone to occur when the skin is thin, or if the tape is applied with too much tension. *Exacting, small-bite, interrupted skin sutures will always give edge-to-edge approximation superior to that obtained with only skin tapes.*

When tapes and sutures are used in combination for skin closure, avoid leaving the skin tapes applied

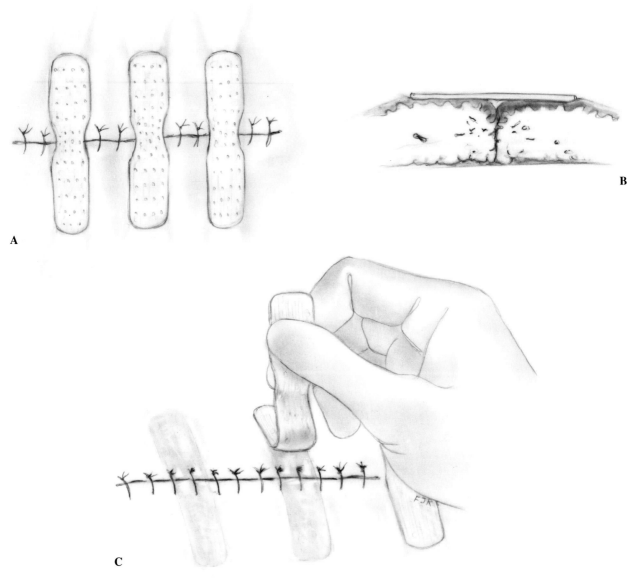

**Figure 7.6**

directly over the sutures for longer than five days. When left for longer periods, the tape imprints the suture mark into the skin and may leave a permanent scar. Removal of adhesive tape in contact with an underlying suture will be uncomfortable as it adheres to the suture and pulls it upward. This may be avoided by cutting the suture to release it from the skin when lifting of the tape first starts to elevate the loop.

An elastic strip has the advantages of being able to expand slightly when wound edema occurs after 24 to 48 hours, and then to draw the skin edges into closer approximation as the swelling subsides. It is a common error to apply an elastic skin tape under excessive stretch or tension. This will result in a blister or "shear burn" of the skin at the points of attachment. In Figure 7.6C skin tapes are being removed at the fifth day after surgery. The red and blistered areas under each area of fixation represent shear injuries of the skin. They indicate that the tape was applied with excessive tension. This is an avoidable complication.

A second cause of redness and dermatitis under skin strips may be skin hypersensitivity to an ingredient in the adhesive used on the tape. The incidence of such allergies is low, but the possibility must be kept in mind. Tapes should be removed quickly and the skin well cleaned at the first suggestion of redness or itching. When tapes are removed early for any reason, it is a comfort if skin sutures have also been used as they will provide continuing security of the wound closure.

One of the most useful applications of sterile adhesive tapes is in the closure of lacerations in the emergency room. After the wound has been cleaned and its extent diagnosed, many lacerations may be effectively drawn together by the use of butterfly dressings or multiple adhesive skin tapes. These may be applied without the use of any anesthetic. This is especially valuable in treating frightened children who may have other injuries. It also avoids the use of foreign bodies in contaminated wounds and does not run the risk of leaving any suture or hatchmarks in skin. In areas such as the face, scars from wide suture marks are common after repairs of lacerations in the emergency room. They often require later surgical excision and the need to excise much valuable skin at the time of a scar revision.

How much better to get primary wound closure with skin tapes! Often the healing will be surprisingly satisfactory and no late scar revision may be needed. This is especially true if the original laceration was parallel to a line of skin relaxation.

When the healing is less than perfect, scar revision may take place with a sedated and psychologically prepared child, the surgery is "clean" and unlikely to result in a wound infection, and the plastic surgeon will have minimum scarring of the original tissues. This provides the optimum opportunity to minimize tension on the healing scar and obtain optimum repair.

**The Logan bow**

At times an external dressing technique can be used to reduce tension not only on a skin closure but also on deep closure of muscles and fascia.

The Logan bow (Fig. 7.7A) is a useful special application of this concept. The Logan bow is a U-shaped metal bar with loops and hooks at each end to allow attachment of two strips of adhesive tape. As shown in Figure 7.7B, two 4-inch-long strips of 1-inch-wide adhesive tape are cut, and 1 inch of tape is folded back on itself to provide each strip with a nonsticky adjustable tab. This folded end may be trimmed slightly to make it fit easily into the metal loop at each end of the Logan bow. The sharp metal prongs on each loop are then pressed through the tape tabs to secure the tape strips to the bow and fix their lengths.

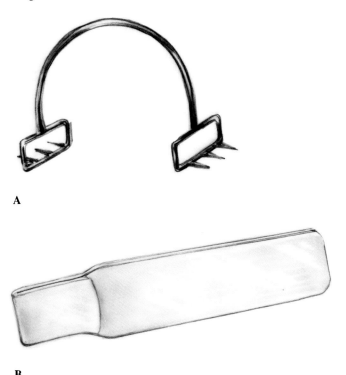

A

B

**Figure 7.7**

The bow is now ready for application across the wound. It may be used in many parts of the body, but its most common application is to fix the two sides of the upper or lower lip together after injury or surgical repair following treatment of congenital or neoplastic defects.

In Figure 7.7C the Logan bow has been applied to a full-thickness wound of the upper lip. The muscles, vermilion, and skin are first sutured. A skin protectant such as compound tincture of benzoin or Mastisol is then painted on the skin of each cheek and allowed to dry. The cheeks are then each pulled toward the midline by the operator a sufficient distance to remove all muscle and skin tension on the suture line. This position will usually cause a fold along each nasolabial crease. With the cheeks held in this position, the adhesive parts of the tapes on each side of the Logan bow are applied to the face. The tension is checked and may be increased or decreased on one or both sides by resetting the tabs on the sharp hooks on each loop of the bow.

This device is quite effective in controlling the facial muscles so that talking, eating, or laughing will not exert undesirable pull on the lip closure.

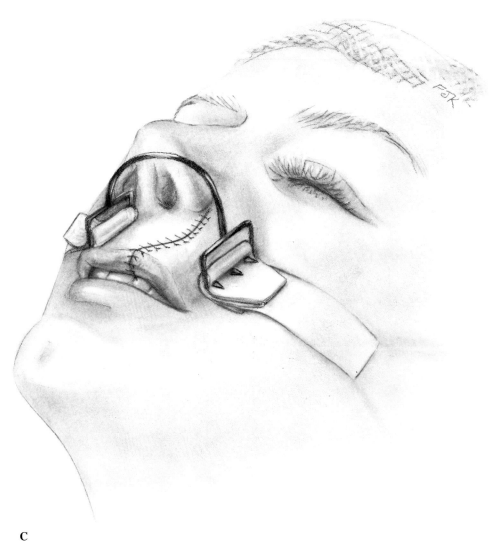

C

**Figure 7.7**

The elevated arch of the metal bow also allows the nursing staff or the patient to keep the suture line clean during the postoperative period. An ordinary dressing in this area tends to collect moisture, saliva, and food, making it wet and uncomfortable, as a result of eating and the presence of oral and nasal secretions.

In small children, the bow should be left in place for some days after the lip sutures have been removed. It will provide useful protection should the child move, cry, or fall during that time.

## Pressure Dressings

### Nonelastic dressings

Very few soft dressings are capable of providing meaningful pressure to a wound in the postoperative period.

In the 1940s Vilray Blair, in studies at Washington University, applied plaster casts to the outside of various types of pressure dressings that had been made from sponges, cotton mechanic's waste, and bandage and applied to the head and neck, the extremities, or to the chest. He included air bulbs within these dressings and used a manometer to monitor the actual pressure exerted by the dressings during the hours following surgery. Not surprisingly, he found that even very firmly wrapped bandages became quickly compressed and packed by patient movements. There was little remaining pressure under any of these bandages within 20 minutes after application.

Surgeons should not delude themselves into thinking that they can use gauze and tape to provide meaningful pressure on a postoperative wound. Nevertheless, if pressure on a skin surface can be maintained above that of the level within the venous capillaries and below the level of the systolic arterial pressure, control of edema and enhanced healing may result. To achieve such results with dressing techniques, special equipment is required.

### Elastic dressings

If elastic dressing materials are put under sufficient stretch or compression, it is possible to provide continuing postoperative pressure on wounds. Ace bandages are commonly used for this purpose. Extremities, faces, and chests are often wrapped with Ace bandages to maintain pressure.

But beware! *These efforts to apply pressure on a wound have produced far more harm than good.*

The use of Ace bandages is associated with significant danger. In most instances, with movements of the patient, the wrappings become loose within a few hours. This is probably a blessing, as loose bandages do little harm in most circumstances. In such cases it would have been less expensive—and the dressings would have remained more secure and professional in appearance—had simple roller bandages and tape been used instead.

When elastic bandages are wrapped more tightly and secured more effectively, the dangers increase. It is difficult for even an experienced surgeon to wrap an Ace bandage with just the proper amount of tension to benefit wound healing. If it is even a little too tight, discomfort, reduced blood flow, and joint stiffness may occur. As edema develops in the first days after surgery, the tightness increases and even more circulatory problems may ensue. *The risk of using an elastic wrap will almost always exceed the theoretical gain.*

By the same token, surgeons have tried incorporating sea sponges or compressible blocks of synthetic plastic materials in dressings. These materials have been used to replace the cotton and gauze that are more commonly used to form tie-on bolus dressings when fixing skin grafts in place. The continuing expansile force exerted by these elastic materials against the confining sutures would often pull the sutures through the wound margins, thus defeating the purpose of the bolus.

Most experienced surgeons now realize the positive value and safety of dressings that gradually compact and spontaneously reduce the pressure they exert on the wound. The true pressure dressing is rarely indicated, and elastic materials are not appropriate for most surgical dressings.

## Dressings for Psychological or Aesthetic Needs

Some surgical dressings are used primarily to prevent the patient or others from seeing the recent surgical wound.

Even well-performed operations that are healing nicely may sometimes create enough deformity to produce unfavorable reactions when viewed by a layman. This is particularly true of operations about the eyes or face, about the external genitalia, or involving the hands. Sutures, oozing blood, open wounds, temporarily displaced anatomy, or fresh skin grafts may cause distress, anxiety, and continued questioning of the surgeon if left uncovered.

A simple covering bandage over such areas will

spare any patient considerable embarrassment and explanation.

Certain patients are so constituted psychologically that one may predict an extraordinary degree of anxiety about their healing. The surgeon will minimize that concern and improve the patients' state of mind if such wounds are kept discreetly covered until the initial phases of healing have occurred.

## Drains

### Differing Views

Surgeons have always disagreed about when they need to use drains. Some like to drain every wound—clean or contaminated, wet or dry. Others resist the use of drains unless they are dealing with an established infection or they find that they are totally unable to obtain effective hemostasis in a wound before closing it. The ideal lies somewhere in between these two approaches. The decision in each case should be based on known surgical principles.

### Reasons for Draining a Wound

*A drain is used only to allow continuing escape from a wound of fluid that is better outside than left within the wound.*

The fluids in question include frank pus, exudates containing inflammatory bacteria (from a contaminated wound), blood, lymph, urine, bile, saliva, or other contents of the gastrointestinal tract. The aqueous material of the anterior chamber of the eye and cerebrospinal fluid are examples of body fluids that are rarely deliberately drained to an outside surface of the body.

When drains are used in infected or contaminated wounds, they should be left in place long enough (5 to 7 days) to establish a sinus track. This track should remain open as long as needed to prevent any reaccumulation and further trapping of fluids and bacteria within the tissues. Premature drain removal may be followed by healing of the skin and the development of a deep abscess.

### Management of Postoperative Hematoma

Perhaps the single most common reason for draining wounds is to avoid the development of a postoperative wound hematoma. Small amounts of clot in a wound will be slowly absorbed by the body, but the breakdown of red blood cells and the release of hematin and other products cause much injury to the healing wound. Thin overlying flaps of skin may even develop necrosis and gangrene if a significant amount of blood is left beneath them.

The removal of any significant amount of liquid or clotted blood from a wound *as soon as possible* is an excellent axiom for any surgeon. Aspiration of hematomas by needle (#18 or #17 gauge) is notoriously ineffective. If a drain was not used at the time of surgery, and a hematoma develops, prompt reopening of a part of the wound and insertion of a sterile grooved director will usually be of great assistance.

In Figure 7.8 a hematoma has been discovered in a "clean" surgical wound 3 days after surgery. A suture has been removed from one end of the incision, and a sterile grooved director has been inserted until its tip reaches the center of the hematoma. A firm rolling motion of a sponge directs the blood toward the opening in the incision. This motion is repeated patiently until all vestiges of liquid or clotted blood are expressed. If any continued or fresh oozing of bright red blood is seen at the end of this process, it is usually wise to replace the grooved director with a sterile rubber drain of appropriate length.

### When to Drain

As a general principle, when in doubt, the surgeon should choose to drain the wound. There are very few drawbacks to the use of a drain. If it proves to have been unnecessary, very little additional scarring or discomfort will have resulted. For years surgeons hesitated to use prophylactic drains in clean wounds. They feared the possible retrograde entry of bacteria along the open track of the drain. Numerous laboratory studies and clinical observations have showed this concern to be unwarranted. We now recognize that virtually *every surgical wound is already contaminated with bacteria at the time of closure.* The old idea that we were able to maintain absolute asepsis in the operating room has been shown to be misguided. A critical mixture of bacterial dose and a vulnerable surgical wound are both needed before clinical wound sepsis develops.

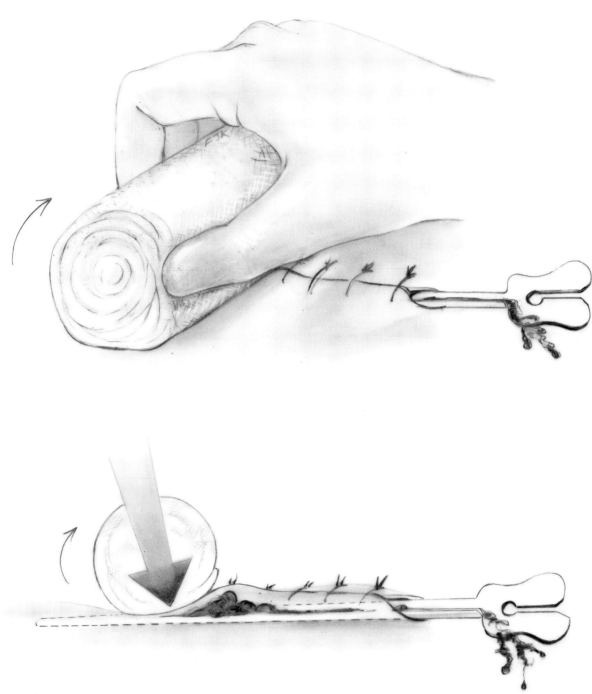

**Figure 7.8**

The bacterial dose becomes more dangerous as its quantity ($>10^3$ organisms per gram of tissue) and pathogenicity increase, but if the surgical wound is free of necrotic tissue, dead space, and blood clot, and if all remaining tissue has a healthy circulation, few established wound infections will result.

Surgeons have learned that the best way to reduce the incidence of wound infections is to *improve their handling of tissue and leave well-vascularized wounds with good natural defenses and no food material (blood or gangrenous tissue) for the inevitably present bacteria.* If the surgeon does not put the body at too great a disadvantage, the wonderful mechanism of leukocyte phagocytosis joins with other host defenses to eliminate bacteria and handle the healing problems.

*When surgical infections occur we must usually blame the surgeon—and not the bacteria!* Drains will rarely introduce infection into a wound that was otherwise destined to heal per primam. Again, *when in doubt, drain!*

## Open Versus Closed Drainage

### Open drainage

Traditional open drainage of a surgical wound consists of inserting a nonadherent (rubber or plastic) strip of material into the deepest recess of the wound. The drain must be long enough to extend beyond the skin surface.

Figure 7.9 shows a rubber drain that has been placed in a wound. The end of the drain has been allowed to emerge at one angle of the surgical incision as closure proceeds. A single suture has been placed through both the drain and the skin margin to prevent accidental displacement of the former. The ends of this suture and excess length of the drain are about to be cut off with the scissors. By cutting this suture the same length as the exposed end of the drain, the surgeon will find it easy to identify and cut the correct suture at the time of drain removal. Note that a "delayed" suture has been placed across the skin margins on either side of the drain. Initially, this suture is tied with a large loose loop and folded into the dressing. When the drain is removed after a few days, this loop is cut near the knot and a clamp is used to tie a knot that will close the skin incision at the site of drain removal. This technique of delayed suturing eliminates depressed puckering of the scar in that part of the incision (often seen if the drainage site is allowed to heal spontaneously).

### Closed suction drainage

Closed drainage differs from open drainage in two respects: First, the skin of the incision (or of a separate stab wound for the drain) is secured tightly around the emerging drain. This fit must be snug enough to prevent any gross air leak. In addition, the drain itself must have a wall of sufficient thickness that it will not collapse if suction is placed on its lumen.

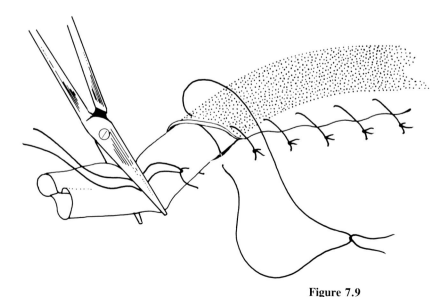

**Figure 7.9**

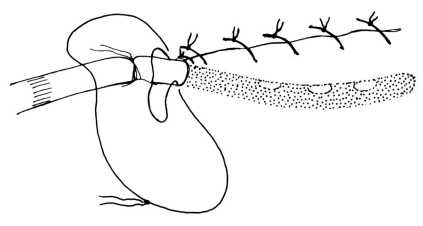

**Figure 7.10A**

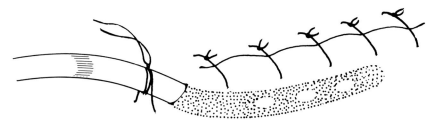

**Figure 7.10B**

Figure 7.10*A* shows a closed drainage system. A plastic catheter with several perforations near its tip has been placed beneath the full length of an incision. The catheter emerges through the angle of the skin incision. The sutures close the skin around the catheter snugly enough to prevent an air leak when suction is applied. In some instances a small separate stab wound may be used for this purpose, as in Figure 7.10*B*. The catheter is routinely sutured to the skin, and a delayed suture with a large loop is placed to complete closure of the incision at the time of catheter removal.

When suction is applied to the end of a closed drainage system, blood and fluid will be evacuated from the wound, and atmospheric pressure will tend to collapse any dead space beneath the skin. Closed suction in this manner may be continued for days, or until the return of fluids through the catheter becomes inconsequential.

At times a suction catheter will become blocked with clots. It may be necessary to flush fluid back into the wound to reopen the catheter. If one is unsuccessful in opening the catheter and re-establishing the suction, the catheter should be removed. A plugged catheter will do more harm than good if left in place and allowed to block the exit of blood and fluid. Suction drains may be used with ambulatory patients if they are instructed in the method of emptying the suction bulb so as to maintain cleanliness, while maintaining negative pressure.

## Suture Removal

### Techniques of Suture Removal

Suture removal continues to be an important aspect of surgical technique. Most patients have some dread of suture removal, especially if they have never had sutures removed, or if they experienced the discomfort of having sutures removed by a rough or impatient surgeon.

In adults, suture removal should always be painless. The technique should concentrate on *not* pulling on any part of the suture until its loop has been divided.

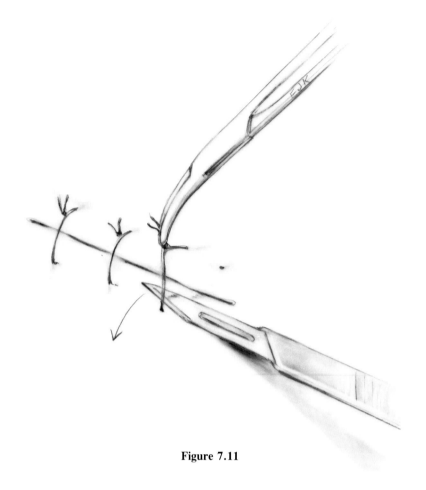

**Figure 7.11**

**Removing interrupted sutures**

When the short ends of a simple suture are lifted with a clamp in preparation for its removal, the lifting should be gentle and the suture should not tug on the skin until the tip of the scissors or the edge of a #11 knife blade has clipped the loop. If the suture bites are extremely small, the surgeon should use a bright light and a pair of binocular magnifying lenses to improve visibility. It is wise to clean any crusts from the suture line with 3% hydrogen peroxide solution before starting.

Figure 7.11 shows an effective method of removing fine sutures with a #11 knife blade. The knife tip is slipped gently under the suture loop, which is cut with a single slow, sawing stroke. The clamp on the short ends of the suture is used only to give counterforce to any outward push produced by the sawing knife blade. The suture should be cut as closely as possible to the point where it emerges from the skin on the side of the incision opposite the knot. In Figure 7.11, a suture has already been cut and the surgeon

is using his knife blade to put counter force against the skin as the clamp gently extracts the remaining suture material. This allows the surgeon to draw the minimum length of exposed and possibly contaminated suture material beneath the skin and through the tissues. If scissors are used, they should have at least one very fine pointed tip. Only the very end of this tip should be inserted under the suture loop and the scissors then closed without lifting or stretching the loop upward away from the skin.

The surgeon should be sure that his scissors are sharp and that they cut well at the tips before removing the first suture.

It is considerate if the surgeon will show the patient the first suture he removes. If he has removed it painlessly, the patient will be visibly reassured and will relax for the rest of the removal. This "see how easy it is" demonstration technique is especially effective with young children. In fact, a particularly apprehensive child may be helped to relax if the surgeon will simply cut off a long tail of one suture and

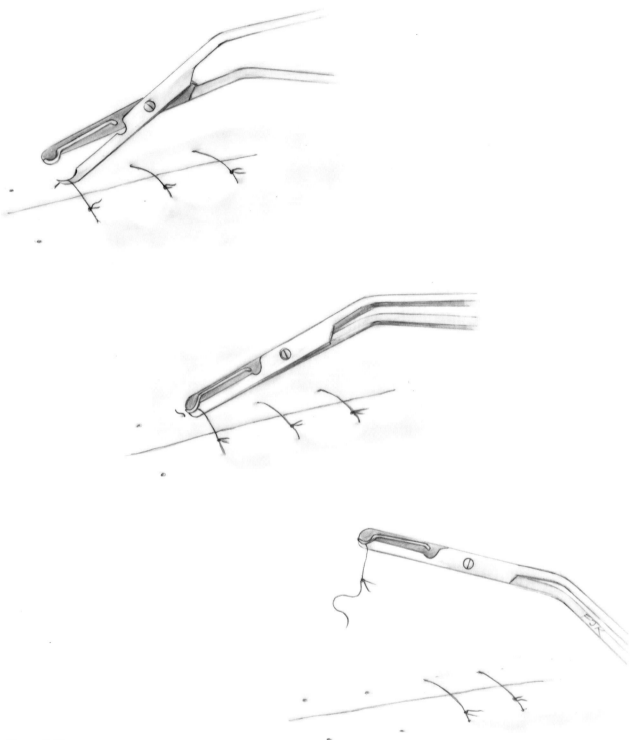

**Figure 7.12**

show it to the child as the first step in removing the stitches.

In all instances, the surgeon should take a seat and not appear to be in any hurry when about to remove stitches.

### Special instruments
If the surgeon has occasion to remove large num-

bers of fine sutures, he may wish to obtain one of the special tools that makes the process easier.

Figure 7.12 shows a tool, the Lashal scissors, that allows the surgeon to cut and grasp a suture with a single motion. This instrument avoids the risk (especially in children) of having the patient move and experience discomfort after a clamp has been placed on the suture ends and before the loop has been divided.

173

When this tool is used, the suture is cut adjacent to the knot, the cut suture is simultaneously clamped and held by the closing special tip (see inset Fig. 7.12). Note that the suture is first clamped by the nose of the instrument, just adjacent to the point where it will be cut. Then further closure and compression of the spring will sever the suture, but leave it firmly held for withdrawal. Some of the exposed loop will be drawn through the deep part of the wound, thus it is best to make the cut quite near the point where the loop of the suture emerges through the skin.

**Removing buried running sutures**

Running intradermal cuticular sutures may be removed with a single slow pull after cutting the suture loop at each end of the incision and after cutting off the knot at *one* end. Prolene and nylon have low coefficients of friction with tissue, and they slide out easily. Other suture materials have greater surface friction and are not as suitable for this technique.

If the surgeon finds that the suture has been placed so that it sticks and does not readily pull out, he should resist the temptation to pull harder and risk having it break off beneath the skin.

Figure 7.13 shows a very useful method for extraction of a ''hung-up'' buried continuous suture that does not slide free when modest traction is applied. A loop is first tied in the exposed end of the suture, and a rubber band is joined to this loop and stretched in the desired direction of pull. While stretched, it is taped to the skin. The entire unit may be covered with a light dressing and the patient is sent home. The band will slowly extract the balky suture over the next one or two hours.

When a continuous suture is not buried, every third or fourth loop can be snipped, and each short segment of suture is then easily withdrawn.

## Timing of Suture Removal

Perhaps the most important rule in selecting the ideal time for suture removal is to factor in the major variables of each particular wound and individualize the removal time indicated by each.

With a few exceptions, sutures should be removed at the earliest time possible without undue risk of wound separation. This means that the surgeon must balance his estimate of the level of wound tensile strength against any ill effects that will occur if the sutures are left in for a longer period.

Sutures that are left too long will cause the skin

to become inflamed, will cut into tissue, cause itching and sepsis, and produce permanent hatch scars. In the skin of the face, sutures left in place longer than five days are likely to cause hatchmark scars.

At five days after surgery, the tensile strength of even a healthy wound is just a fraction of normal skin strength. That tensile strength does not approach normal until approximately 70 days after suturing.

If skin sutures are removed on the fifth day, and the freshly healed unprotected incision is then bumped, scratched, or stretched, it is very likely to disrupt. How may the surgeon reduce this danger and still remove the sutures before they begin to leave telltale scars?

At the time of surgery there are three useful measures that will allow the surgeon to remove sutures safely at an earlier date postoperatively than would otherwise be possible. These are:

1. *Generous undermining and surgical advancement* of tissues will reduce tension at the time of original wound closure.
2. *Internal suturing* of deeper tissue layers may also bring skin edges together and reduce the tension needed for approximation by skin sutures.
3. *External fixation* of skin or joints by taping or casts may be used to supplement the closure of both buried and cuticular sutures.

These three measures are all directed at reducing the load on the skin sutures. This reduces closure tension and improves the circulation. Not only does tensile strength build up more rapidly along a low tension suture line, but there is also less skin separation in the period immediately following suture removal.

## Skin Fixation to Replace Sutures

The danger of wound separation can be further reduced if the surgeon will use some supplementary method of skin fixation immediately after the early removal of sutures. Two common methods are used to substitute skin fixation for the holding power of sutures at the time of their removal.

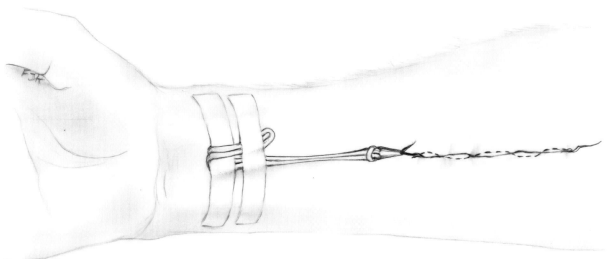

**Figure 7.13**

### Adhesive skin tapes

Rigid skin strips with adhesive backing (Steri-strips) may be applied across an incision for additional security after suture removal.

These strips will hold for a few days, but the secretions and shedding of the skin may make it necessary to replace them frequently (every 4–5 days) if secure support is to be maintained. They tend to be relatively ineffective if applied across a concave surface.

### Collodion gauze patches

If the skin surface is first cleaned carefully with ether (an excellent lipolytic agent) after suture removal, a patch of fine-mesh ordinary roller gauze bandage may be soaked in flexible collodion and applied across the suture line.

A rectangular piece of gauze is first cut (Fig. 7.14A) of proper size so that it will overlap at least 1 inch on either side of the incision. The rectangle is then dipped in a medicine glass containing flexible collodion (Fig. 7.14B). The well-soaked gauze is next applied to the clean dry skin on both sides of the suture line and allowed to dry over a 5-minute period (Fig. 7.14C).

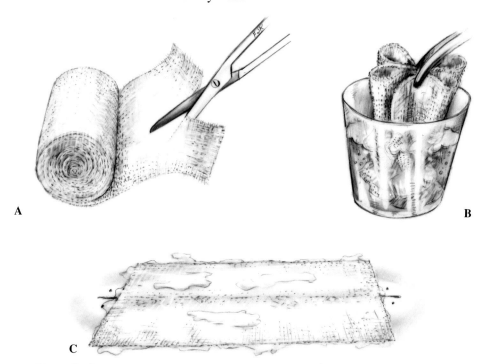

A

B

C

**Figure 7.14**

This patch should be kept dry and it will usually remain quite adherent to the skin for an additional 5 days. At that time it may be removed by the patient. Its edges should be gently peeled off the skin, working toward the incision from either side.

Collodion is well tolerated. The author has never encountered a rash or hypersensitivity in thousands of applications. The splinting and slight stiffness of the skin beneath the collodion patch seem to remind the patient of the still-delicate state of healing and to encourage protection of the area from trauma. The cost of the materials is insignificant.

# 8

# Special Surgical Techniques; Operating Room Hand Signals; The Left-Handed Surgeon

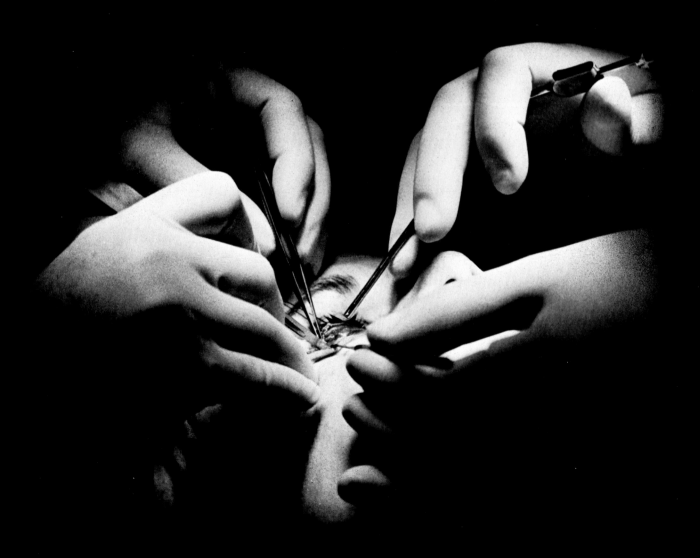

# 8

# Special Surgical Techniques; Operating Room Hand Signals; The Left-Handed Surgeon

## Alloplastic Implants in Surgery

Methylmethacrylate, silicone rubber, and porous Proplast implants are frequently used successfully as substitutes for bone grafts in surgery. Such implants avoid the problems of late bone graft absorption and spare patients the morbidity of donor sites used for harvesting allografts of bone or cartilage.

Although alloplastic implants are incapable of supplying nutrition for bacteria, they may, if improperly inserted, produce surgical wounds with ultrasound mechanics that will favor the growth of bacteria or cause the gradual thinning and breakdown of soft tissues that cover the implants.

This susceptibility to postoperative infections or extrusions has led some surgeons to condemn all implant materials as "foreign bodies" that "cause infections." Some patients are inaccurately told that their failed implants were "rejected by the body." A few surgeons remain adamant in refusing to use such alloplastic materials. Such an extreme view may deny many surgical benefits to their patients.

A review of the laboratory evidence and the experience and published reports of thousands of surgeons over the past four decades indicates that *postoperative problems with surgical implants are largely a matter of failures in surgical technique rather than problems related to the chemical nature of the implant materials.*

Most alloplastic materials that are used in surgery are quite inert and beautifully tolerated by human tissues. When well-fitted and placed deeply in highly vascular areas, they have served well for the remaining lifetimes of thousands of patients.

The surgeon is unwise to extend his indications for using surgical implants by placing them too near the body surface, by covering them with soft tissues of reduced vascularity, or by closing the wound in a way that compresses the soft tissue or deforms a permanently elastic implant. The soft tissue will be made ischemic and damaged by the force of continued implant expansion. The surgeon should not be surprised when a late extrusion or other complication occurs. He should blame himself and not the implant. Figure 8.1 illustrates some of the common surgical errors made when attempting to use a silastic ear framework in external ear reconstruction. Because of the paucity of local skin and its thin and sometimes anesthetic condition, the ear is one of the most difficult areas of the body for the successful use of an implant.

The cross-section of the convoluted elastic silicone rubber framework shows that it has been partly flattened in Figure 8.1 against the mastoid bone to facilitate wound closure. In this wound, there is simply insufficient skin for the surgeon to drape it up and down into direct contact with all the hills and valleys of the external surface of the implant. This skin deficiency thus causes bridging, with resultant dead spaces. Two of these spaces have become filled with serum and blood clots. The lack of sufficient absorptive tissue surfaces about the clots will cause them to linger, and liberated hematin will directly damage the deep surface of the overlying skin.

Meanwhile, the unremitting elasticity of the frame continues to exert pressure upward against the normally thin skin of the ear region. At two points of maximum pressure, the cutaneous blood flow has been seriously slowed, and the skin has become quite thin. If this skin also happens to be anesthetic (as a result of sectioning of the sensory nerves at the time of surgery), its defense against ulceration and implant extrusion is reduced even further.

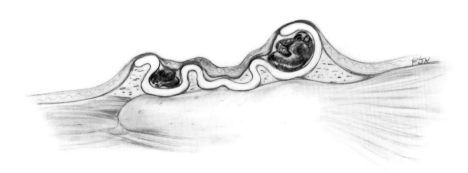

**Figure 8.1**

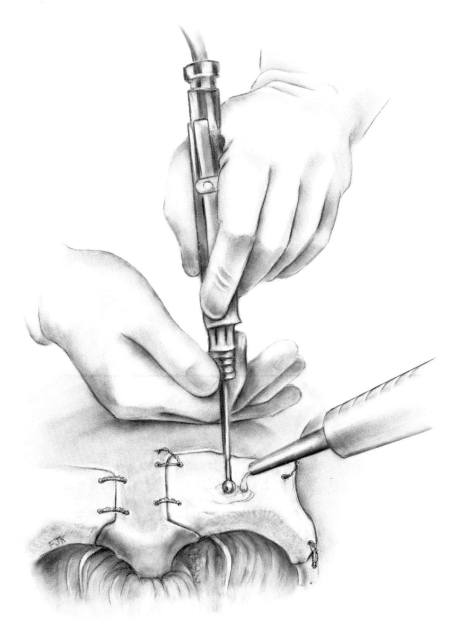

**Figure 8.2**

## Bone Carpentry

Bone and cartilage are living and dynamic tissues. Like soft tissue, they may be injured by rough handling, heat, or desiccation. Bone requires a good blood supply for proper healing. The surgeon who forgets this works on bone at the peril of his patient.

The rigid matrixes of bone and cartilage and the frameworks of some of the dense alloplastic implant materials require surgeons to use special tools that are seldom needed for soft tissue surgery. Sharp periosteal elevators, osteotomes, chisels, mallets, saws, curettes, rongeurs, bone cutters, bone clamps, screws, pins, plates, rods, and wires are all part of that family of special instruments. They are used to expose, cut, shape, clean, or fix fragments of bone and cartilage. The surgical specialty of orthopedics depends heavily upon the skillful use of such tools in skeletal manipulations. Other surgical specialists such as general surgeons, plastic surgeons, neurosurgeons, chest surgeons, and otolaryngologists are also frequently involved in bone carpentry. The ability to properly handle bone and cartilage is an important aspect of basic surgery. Special bone carpentry techniques are important aspects of the work of several surgical specialties.

In recent years, the development of power tools driven by electricity or compressed air has increased

RPMs, improved the torque of drills, and added new capabilities to bone surgery. At the same time, these high-speed saws and drills have introduced new hazards to tissue. These hazards demand that surgeons practice new precautions that have resulted in modifications of some of our surgical techniques.

High-speed drills and saws rapidly generate heat. Heat will kill the osteoblasts in bone lacunae and alter the protein in the adjacent supporting bony matrix. Power tools must be used with a light touch and for brief periods. Cool saline irrigation should be constantly dripped on any bone at the site of contact with the blade or burr.

Figure 8.2 illustrates two autogenous iliac bone grafts that have been shaped and wired with stainless steel wires into defects in each supraorbital ridge region. The two supraorbital nerves were saved and may be seen reflected down with the tissues of the forehead flap and orbit into a protected position. The twisted ends of each of the steel wires have been bent and inserted into one of the drill holes in the recipient bone. One wire has been left unseated to show this method of burying the ends.

The surgeon is using a pneumatic power drill and a round-headed burr to refine the shape of the bone. He is changing the contour by producing a natural concavity just above the ridge of the brow. Note that he holds the drill with *both* hands. It is not possible to position the hand that controls the power switch on the drill handle sufficiently close to the high-speed rotating burr to adequately brace it against a sudden catching of the bit and displacement. A jumping drill can do major damage if its spin catches the adjacent soft tissue. This risk is avoided by the surgeon's use of his second hand to grasp and guide the nose of the drill while bracing the dorsum of the fingers of that hand against the surgical field. The fingers of this bracing hand provides the fine control movements needed to accurately position the drill point as the cutting proceeds.

Whenever a rotating drill point is in contact with bone, the surgical assistant uses an Asepto bulb syringe to gently wet the bone and the spinning drill tip. The tip of the syringe must be placed directly above the area to be kept wet, but it must be located so that *neither the syringe nor the assistant's hand obstructs the surgeon's view of the burr and adjacent bone.* If smoke is seen to arise from the site of the drill or saw, the assistant has failed to do his job, and bone healing will be impaired.

Surgeons have often noted the slow absorption of autogenous bone grafts occurring, sometimes many months after satisfactory uncomplicated initial healing. This is especially true in the case of bone grafts used primarily for contour restoration. In some instances, slow absorption may be related to lack of rigid fixation to adjacent bone. In other cases, the vascularity (and consequent healing capacities) of the recipient bone or of the investing soft tissue may have been below normal. In these circumstances the usual creeping replacement of the graft with osteoblasts that migrate in front adjacent host bone and the gradual remineralization of the graft matrix may not proceed to completion. Graft absorption will follow.

When such delicate mechanisms are involved, it takes little imagination to realize that good surgical technique demands that any existing circulation to bone fragments should be preserved. The *minimal elevation of periosteum and the maintenance of all soft tissue attachments* will do much to improve subsequent bone healing.

Other surgical principles in bone carpentry include exacting fixation of bone to bone and the reapplication of soft tissues so that they coapt closely to bone surfaces and eliminate all dead space. Hematomas that are allowed to form between the surfaces of fracture lines or bone grafts and any adjacent soft tissue will reduce and delay bone revascularization and furnish an excellent food supply for any casual bacteria that may be present.

Six weeks after such an operation the edge of the implant quietly extrudes through the skin. Is such a complication any surprise when so many basic surgical principles have been forgotten or ignored?

Surgeons make a profession out of the successful use of foreign materials inside the human body. Sutures, wires, screws, plates, cerebrospinal fluid shunts, dacron prosthetic vessels, silicone breast implants, lenses for the eye, and artificial hips are but a few of the well-established examples of brilliant long-term successes with the use of alloplastic materials.

The use of implant materials in surgery requires the surgeon to add new principles to his understanding of the needs and architecture of the ideal surgical wound. Once he does so he and his patients will have increasing success with the use of alloplastic materials.

In some cases, surgical implants offer the only hope of improving the quality of life. *Surgical implants are here to stay. They will be used even more frequently in future years.*

## The Removal of "Dog Ears" in Closing Skin

When scars or other dangerous or unsightly lesions are removed surgically, the surgeon will often find, as he closes the wound, that the skin at each end of his incision bunches up above the surface. These little mounds are commonly referred to as "dog ears," for obvious reasons.

When even a small skin lesion is removed by an elliptical excision, dog ears will appear if the surgeon, in his attempt to avoid making a long scar, does not taper the removed ellipsoid gradually. It is far better to make the scar longer than to leave these curious little bumps on each end of the closure. Patients repeatedly confirm that the contour irregularities of a dog ear produce a greater sense of deformity than the increased length of scar that results from its removal.

It is obviously preferable to anticipate and remove potential dog ears at the time of the original surgery. Both patient and surgeon are unhappy about having a second operation to remove them later. They will almost never flatten out spontaneously if they are evident at the end of an operation.

The technique for removing a cutaneous dog ear is straightforward. In Figure 8.3A most of the incision has been closed and a small redundant fold of skin remains. The operator first grasps the center of the fold with his hook and retracts it to one side. He then incises the top surface of the skin fold exactly along the desired line of extension of the closed incision. This cut with the scalpel should begin at the point where the skin fold disappears (flattens) into the surrounding skin and should continue back to join the skin edge of the sutured part of the wound.

Since this skin fold is held only by a single hook, it is rather mobile and sometimes not easy to cut with the knife. If only light pressure is used on the knife blade, the line of cut can be made more accurately. This initial knife cut will incise only the epidermis and partially through the depth of the dermis.

The skin of the dog ear can then be grasped with the forceps (or the hook) as shown in Figure 8.3B, and the scissors used to complete the cut through the remaining deep dermis along the line of the knife cut. The opened flap of dog ear skin is then elevated as shown in Figure 8.3C, and the skin is generously undermined to release all of its attachments to the deep fascia in the immediate area. This will allow the skin to settle into its new position and make the final cut more accurate.

The mobilized and opened flap of skin is then held flat (Fig. 8.3D) so that the excess triangle may be accurately seen and removed by a second cut of the knife. Once again, if the cut is made by stroking back toward the already sutured part of the incision, the skin and knife edge will be more easily controlled. This cut, as before, should include only a portion of the dermis.

In Figure 8.3E the scissors are used to complete the cut of the deep dermis. The shear action of the scissor blades will close off some of the small vessels and result in less skin bleeding than when this cut is completed with a knife. The mobility of this skin fold also makes the use of the scissors more efficient than the scalpel in completing the skin cuts.

The final suturing is then completed (Fig. 8.3F). Note the use of the closed forceps as a simple "pusher" to fix the skin so that the needle tip emerges exactly at the desired point. This "push" technique causes less tissue injury than does grasping the skin with the sharp teeth of the forceps.

This approach to dog ear removal will avoid the need to continue to chase small remaining bumps and buds of skin at wound ends.

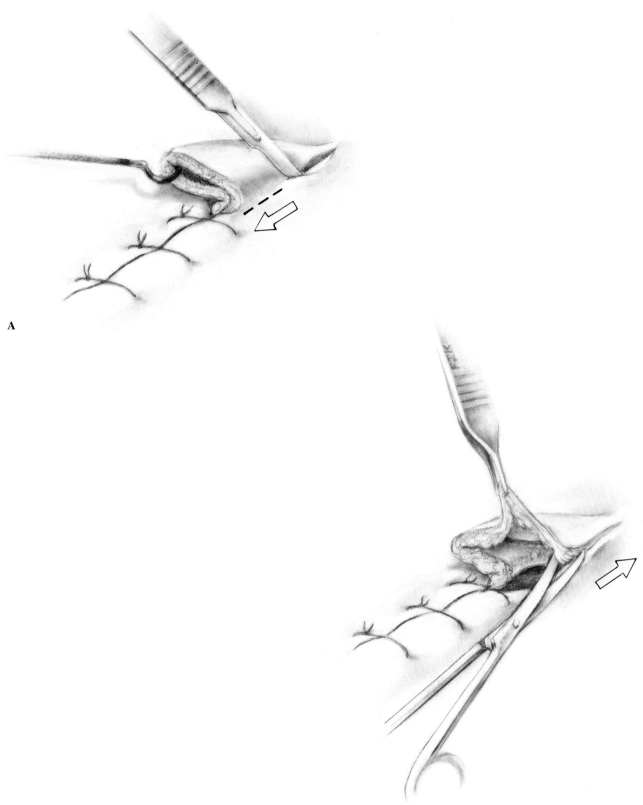

A

B

**Figure 8.3** *(Figure continues)*

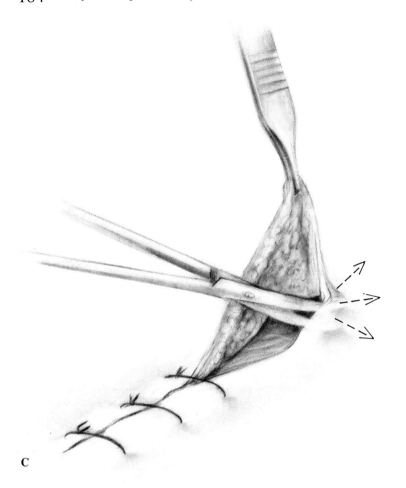

C

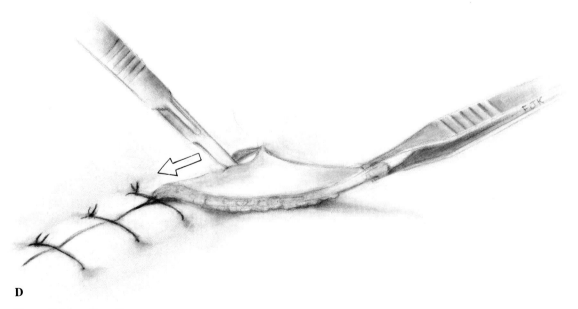

D

**Figure 8.3** *(continued)*

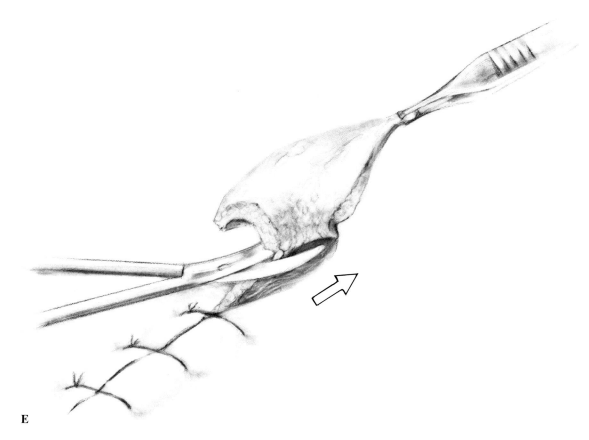

**E**

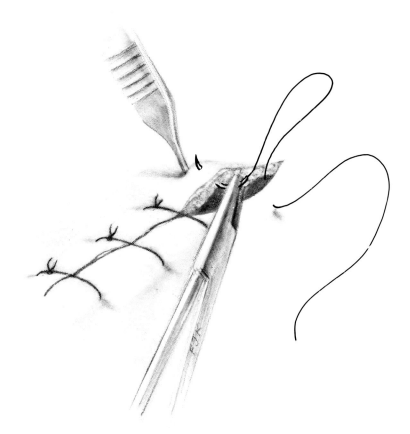

**F**

**Figure 8.3** *(continued)*

## Razabrasion and Dermabrasion

Since the early 1950s, surgeons have used abrasive materials on human skin to smooth irregularities of contour or to remove unsightly or dangerous lesions.

Human skin has surprising toughness. It will withstand considerable trauma and still heal with a uniform surface, as long as the reticular dermal layer is not completely penetrated. This is true of injuries that are chemical, thermal, or mechanical.

Thus, it is often possible to remove scars or lesions in the upper (more superficial) levels of the skin by some form of tangential excision. Chemical peel techniques with phenolic or trichloracetic acids are used by plastic surgeons to remove fine wrinkles in the face. These methods may be painful, they occasionally cause deep burns or thick scars, and they frequently alter the pigment pattern in skin. They should be used with great caution.

Mechanical dermabrasion began with the use of ordinary sandpaper. This abrasive paper was thumb-tacked about wooden blocks, and the patients' faces were rubbed—sometimes for hours to remove scars or the irregularities of acne infections. The process was tedious, and sometimes grains of sand were trapped in the healing skin, but the results were encouraging.

With time, powered instruments using rotating wire brushes replaced the sandpaper. Results improved, but deep cuts with the brushes occurred on some occasions. Wire brushes were gradually replaced with pear-shaped diamond cutting burrs and similar drills.

The softness of living skin makes cutting it with any high-speed burr rather difficult. Blood obscures the depth of cut, and surgeons have turned to temporary freezing of the skin with freon gas to make it firm and to reduce bleeding during the abrading process. The freon was sprayed on the skin to freeze it, and the dermabrasion was then quickly carried out before thawing. The abrasion of frozen skin was more successful, but the technique was awkward and patients objected to the smell of the gas.

In the 1970s, at the University of Virginia, we returned to a more surgical method of tangential excision of skin lesions. This was but a modification of the methods plastic surgeons had used for years to remove split-thickness skin grafts for use in other parts of the body. Vilray Blair had found that a large, very sharp knife blade (Fig. 8.4A) would allow the controlled and uniform removal of skin at almost any thickness (0.008 to 0.036 inch) desired by the surgeon. He used the removed skin for grafting, but the same principle is of value for the debridement of burn eschars, or for the removal or smoothing out of undesirable lesions. The technique for removing skin with a long-bladed, stiff backed blade is described in Chapter 1.

We have coined the term "razabrasion" to describe a method of using a thin sharp razor to facilitate the removal of scars, pits, creases, or lesions that occupy only part of the thickness of the skin. On flat surfaces, a straight-edged razor may be used, but if the skin surface is curved, the cutting blade may need a similar curve to remove the lesion evenly. The thin double-edged commercial razor blade is ideal for this purpose. It is very sharp and its blade may be readily bent by the surgeon's fingers. Figure 8.4B shows the best method for holding the blade. The amount of curve may be changed as the cutting proceeds so that the technique of altering the shape of the blade allows it to be used in recesses or valleys. The rotary motion of the wrist allows the blade to move back and forth parallel along a curved plane to the curve of the blade.

Razabrasion allows more accurate control of depth of cutting than does dermabrasion with rotary power tools. It is faster, quieter, and more pleasant for the patient; it produces a biopsy specimen when needed; and it is obviously more gentle on the remaining skin than is dermabrasion. The surface heals in 6 to 10 days.

Thus, razabrasion is a valuable new surgical technique that may largely replace dermabrasion for many types of tangential skin excisions.

## Pinch Testing for Motor Nerve Identification

Surgeons depend on an exacting knowledge of anatomy to avoid injury to vital or important structures when dissecting tissue. At times deformities or disease processes will displace or alter structures so that they have little resemblance to normal, and all fascial planes may become obliterated. Simple methods that aid in the identification of structures are of great value in such circumstances. It is important to protect motor nerves such as the facial, the spinal accessory, and the hypoglossal nerves. The simple pinch test, properly used, is of great value at such times.

Expensive and elaborate nerve stimulators have been designed for motor nerve identification during surgery. Although useful, most electrical stimulators

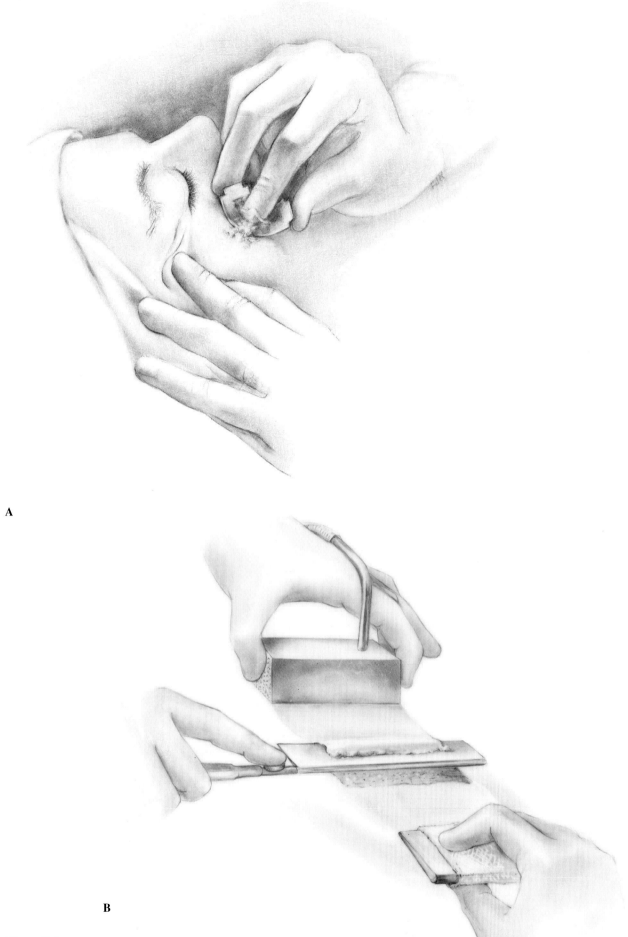

**A**

**B**

**Figure 8.4**

have problems. The electrical current will frequently spread through nearby tissue and stimulate the nerve, even when the probe tip is not exactly localized on the nerve at that moment. This imprecise localization may make division of that adjacent fascia worrisome. At other times, power failure, poor contacts, or grounding problems may cause a false-negative response when a nerve is tested—with disastrous consequences.

All of these problems may be avoided if the surgeon relies on the simple, mechanical, motor nerve pinch test. He must first ascertain that the anesthesiologist is using no muscle paralyzing agents. He must also be sure that his surgical field is draped so that he can readily observe the slightest movement of the muscles innervated by the motor nerve in question.

As the dissection proceeds, the surgeon gently tests any questionable tissue by compressing it with the tips of a small clamp or a smooth-jawed forceps. As he does so he directs an assistant to monitor the muscles supplied by that nerve for any contractions. As he pinches the tissue he asks the assistant, "Any response?" The assistant, without moving his eyes from the muscle area, responds either "twitch" or "no twitch." If the response is "no twitch," the surgeon then slowly increases the force of the clamping while the assistant continues to watch the muscle for any response. If there is none, the surgeon removes the clamp and *cuts only the clamped tissue without ever having removed his eyes from the field*. Over the past three decades, I have found this method of testing for motor nerves 100% reliable. It is rapid, precise, and accurate, and requires no technology that may go astray.

When used with a light touch, the potential for multiple restimulations of the same nerve is present. Continual restimulation of a motor nerve by either electrical or mechanical means will ultimately produce fatigue or poor response; hence, once identified, the nerve should be left as untraumatized as possible.

The pinch test is an invaluable technique for motor nerve identification in surgery; but it must be executed properly!

## Injection Techniques With Local Anesthesia

When patients not under general anesthesia are injected with various solutions, suspensions, and medications, their memory of this experience later will depend largely on the art and skill of the doctor or nurse who does the injection. Technique is paramount. To a large extent, good injection techniques reflect the ability of the injector to imagine and anticipate the anxieties and sensations of the patient. If he empathizes accurately with the patient, he may greatly ameliorate many of the unpleasant aspects of needles and drugs that cause pain or burning sensations.

When approaching an injection, the surgeon must never appear to be hurried. He should move and talk slowly and specifically reassure the patient about the injection. If he deliberately avoids the subject, the patient's worst fears will mount and anxiety will increase.

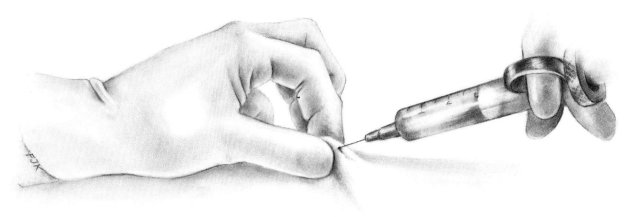

**Figure 8.5**

If the patient is in a position where he cannot see the needle or the surgeon's hands while the skin is being prepped and the syringe is filled, it is only kind to advise him, "I will let you know before I inject anything." This will keep the patient from tensing up prematurely. Most will express their appreciation for this courtesy.

The choice of words when injecting local anesthesia is important. The patient should be told that he will feel a "pinprick." Avoid the words "needle" and "stick." The point of needle entry should be identified for the patient by touching it. Discomfort will be reduced if this area is then pinched firmly between the thumb and index finger of the surgeon's nondominant hand for several seconds before the injection (Figure 8.5). A warning—"You will now feel a little prick"—should be issued to the patient just 2 to 3 seconds before the needle tip enters (and *not* 10 to 20 seconds before).

When a patient is not sedated, the needle should be pushed through the skin quickly and a drop of anesthetic quickly released. Almost all local anesthetic solutions have a very low pH. This acidity of the solution accounts for much of the burning sensation experienced when anesthetic solution first contacts the tissues.

A great deal of this unpleasant sensation can be avoided if a small amount (10 mg/100 ml) of sodium bicarbonate solution is added to the lidocaine anesthetic as the solution is prepared for the syringe. Sodium bicarbonate should not be added to solutions of marcaine as it tends to precipitate this agent out of solution and may result in areas of prolonged (many weeks) skin numbness.

Further reduction in the pain of injection is obtained if the surgeon will continue to inject a drop of fluid ahead of his needle tip, pause 1 to 2 seconds, and then advance his needle into the fluid after some numbing has resulted. He then injects another drop forward, pauses, and advances the needle once again.

When a surgeon is injecting local anesthetic into an already heavily sedated patient, it may be counterproductive to attempt arousal of the patient at the moment of injection. In such instances, the surgeon, without announcement, will simply pinch the skin at the site of injection and insert the needle very slowly through the dermis, attempting to inject the first of the anesthetic without drawing attention to the moment of entry.

In all cases use of a fine (#30 gauge) needle, with silicone coating, will greatly minimize needle pain.

Whenever solutions are injected, it is important that the needle be introduced into the skin at an angle that is tangential to nearby vital structures. If this is done, any sudden lurch or unexpected movement of the patient will not cause the needle to perforate an organ or cause it to penetrate some area of adjacent, nonanesthetized skin.

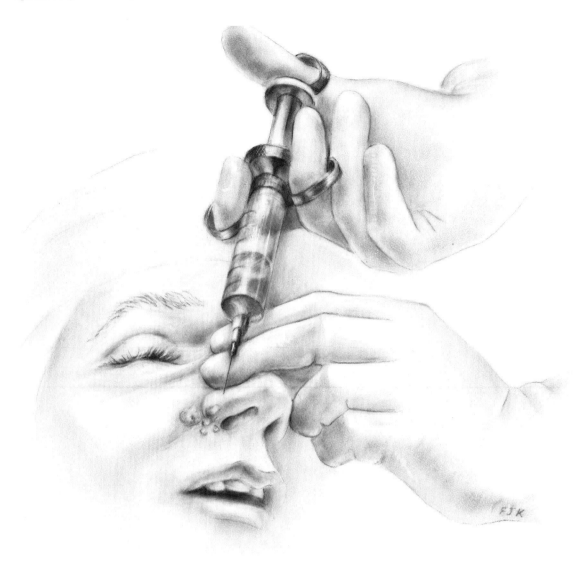

**Figure 8.6**

Figure 8.6 shows a proper technique for injecting the right alar base of the nose. The needle tip is directed away from the eye and at a 45° angle with the surface of the alar skin. The surgeon is using the long and index fingers of his left hand to stabilize the barrel of the syringe in relation to the patient's head. He rests the butt of the needle and the tip of the syringe on these fingers, so that the right hand can be more relaxed and concentrated on the ideal rate of injection of the anesthetic.

When using needles, the surgeon must never forget that *unhurried gentleness, appropriate warnings,* and *patience in waiting for the anesthesia to take effect* are noticed and appreciated by all patients.

## The Left-Handed Surgeon

Many surgeons are dominantly left-handed. In fact, the specialty of plastic surgery has a large (25% to 30%) number of left-handed operators. The exact reason why many left-handed surgeons choose a career in plastic surgery is not yet known. It may be that left-handedness in childhood forces the individual to translate or "mirror" many of the actions of his right-handed friends and teachers. This training may develop an appreciation for symmetry and skill in spatial translations that later attract that individual to choose a field of medicine that lays much emphasis on morphology and symmetry. Neurophysiological studies have shown that the right side of the human brain seems to be responsible for our creative or artistic qualities. Since left-handed people have right brain dominance, this may correlate with the interest of left-handed surgeons in aesthetic and morphologic activities.

Yet all surgeons must develop many skills with both hands. Surgery is truly a *bi*manual profession. The movements of the nondominant hand in using the forceps are just as complex and require as much practice and skill as those of the dominant hand that wields the scissors to cut the tissue that is lifted and presented by those forceps.

In Chapter 1, the right-handed design of most scissors was described. The catches and clasps of surgical clamps are designed for easy release by the right hand, and require "reverse" actions by the thumb and fingers of the left hand.

Left-handed scissors and clamps and needle holders have been designed, but they have never been very popular. The left-handed surgeon has had so many years of childhood practice with tools made for right-handed people that he feels no disadvantage when using right-handed surgical instruments. If the left-handed surgeon also happens to be a teacher of surgery, he may even wish to take advantage of that fact by letting his right-handed residents-in-training stand on the side of the operating table that they will later choose when they are the chief surgeons. This allows them to palpate and observe the operation, just as they will in future years when they are acting as chief surgeons.

When a right-handed surgeon is acting as a first assistant for a left-handed surgeon, naturally he will alter the usual positions of his hands in pulling needles through the tissues. Such adaptations are obvious and only tend to improve everyone's overall surgical dexterity.

The left-handed doctor should have no hesitancy in choosing a career in surgery.

## Hand Signals in the Operating Room

The ideal operating room is a quiet room! Some sounds from the anesthetic gas machines and the equipment monitoring the patient's vital functions are usually evident and necessary. Unfortunately, in recent years, there has been a steady creep of unnecessary noise into the surgical theaters. Additional people (nursing aides, students of anesthesia, messengers from labs or the blood bank) all add more decibels. The operating room intercom calls for an attendant, equipment is dropped, buckets are kicked, the sterilizer cycle completes and its bell begins to ring. The resident's beeper goes off beneath his scrub gown, the nurses loudly count sponges or needles in synchrony, and even—heaven forbid!—a wall telephone in the sterilizer room rings with some trivial message from a ward.

All of this is superimposed on any necessary discussion about the operation between the surgeon and his assistant. At times there will be a loud and prolonged discussion of respiratory physiology between the anesthesiologist and his junior assistant.

Many operations will not prosper or move as smoothly if this background noise is present. Good surgical decisions often require concentration. The human mind has been shown to be much better at concentration in a quiet environment. If we become "noisy-sloppy" in the operating room, our patients will suffer.

Noise reduction and control become even more important in the operating room when the patient is awake and under local anesthesia. In such circumstances, the patient's auditory system is acutely tuned in. All sounds appear to be magnified. Comments by the surgical team are frequently misinterpreted and result in patient fright and anxiety. Words like "Oops!" or "No!" and phrases like "That's bad" or "I don't like that" sound devastating to the patient. The surgical team must have the empathy to imagine how they would react to the words and sounds heard in the operating room.

## "Clamp"

One useful technique to reduce noise and patient anxiety in the operating room is the use of appropriate hand signals by the surgeon and his assistant.

Simple and easily understood motions of the hands have emerged over the years as highly efficient methods of communication between the surgeons and the scrub nurse. These motions allow the surgeon to keep his eyes focused on the brightly illuminated surgical field and tell his assistant just how he might wish to be helped. The scrub nurse should familiarize herself with these simple signals and their meanings. It goes without saying that she must try to keep her eyes on the surgical field and the surgeon's hands, if she is ever to become a first-rate professional. She should look at the back table or the circulating nurse as little as possible and only for brief moments.

When the surgeon extends his opened hand (Fig. 8.7A) without comment he expects his scrub nurse to pass the handle of an artery clamp (or a Kelly clamp if working with larger vessels) into his palm with a distinct "pop" (Fig. 8.7B). He should not have to take his eyes away from the field to know that he has this clamp in his grasp. Thus, the hand signal for a clamp is the simple open hand with extended fingers as shown in Figure 8.7A.

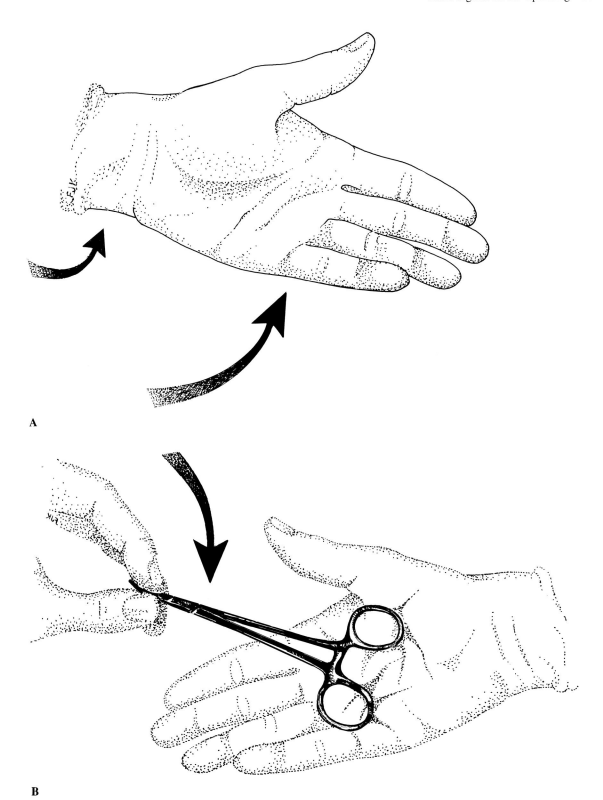

A

B

**Figure 8.7**

## "Forceps"

When the surgeon uses the forceps in his left hand, he holds it as shown in Figure 8.8A. He controls the opening and closing of the forceps with his thumb and index finger. Thus, the common hand signal to request a pair of forceps is a repeated opening and closing of the thumb and fingers to simulate the actions of the forceps. This hand signal is illustrated in Figure 8.8B–C. It may be made with either hand.

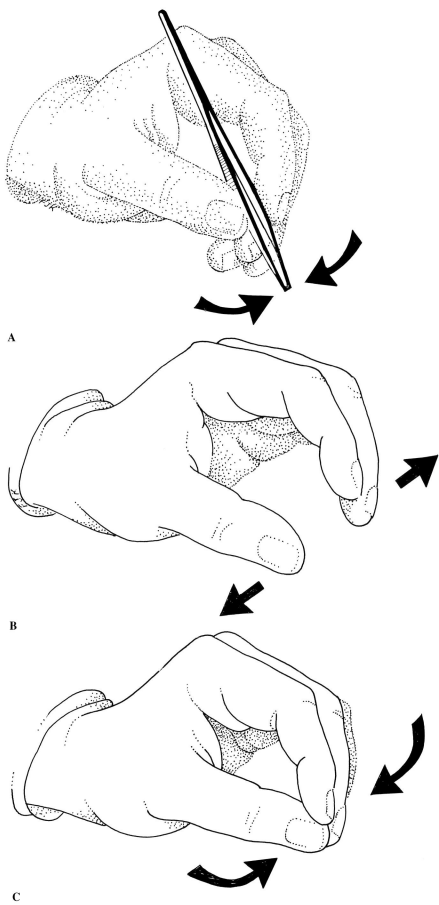

A

B

C
Figure 8.8

195

## "15 Blade"

When doing fine work with a scalpel, the surgeon holds the knife as shown in Figure 8.9*A*. The blade is moved through the tissues by a flexing of the index finger and thumb while the hand is steadied by the contact of the ring and little fingers with the patient. Thus, the hand signal to request a small (#15) bladed scalpel is a repetition of this flexing of the thumb and index finger while their tips are held together as if holding an imaginary knife. This motion is shown in Figure 8.9*B–C*. It is combined with a short forward-and-backward motion of the entire hand and forearm to suggest drawing the knife through the tissues.

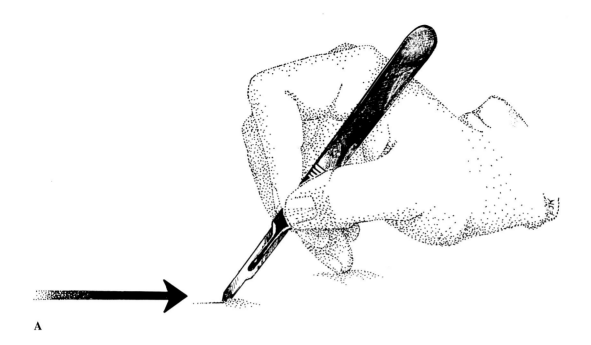

**A**

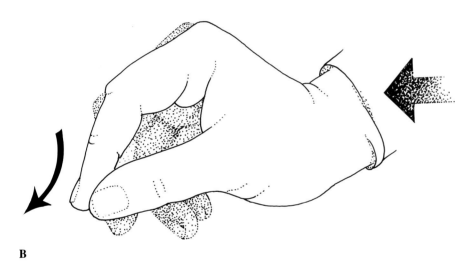

**B**

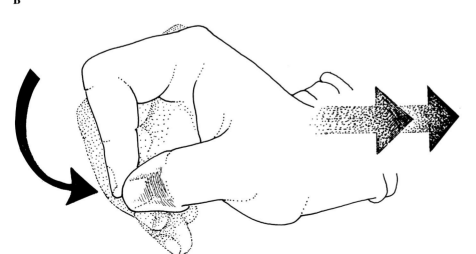

**C**

**Figure 8.9**

## "20 Blade"

When a surgeon uses a large scalpel blade for heavier work, he holds the knife in a power grip as shown in Figure 8.10A. The heads of his metacarpals provide the hand area that provides downward pressure on the blade. The hand signal (Fig. 8.10B–C) for the large knife is thus a short back-and-forth motion of the flexed fingers with an extended wrist. The motion pretends that the knife is held in the hand and resembles the motion of the "bow" hand of a violinist. The pulp of the thumb is pressed in a key pinch against the radial side of the flexed index finger.

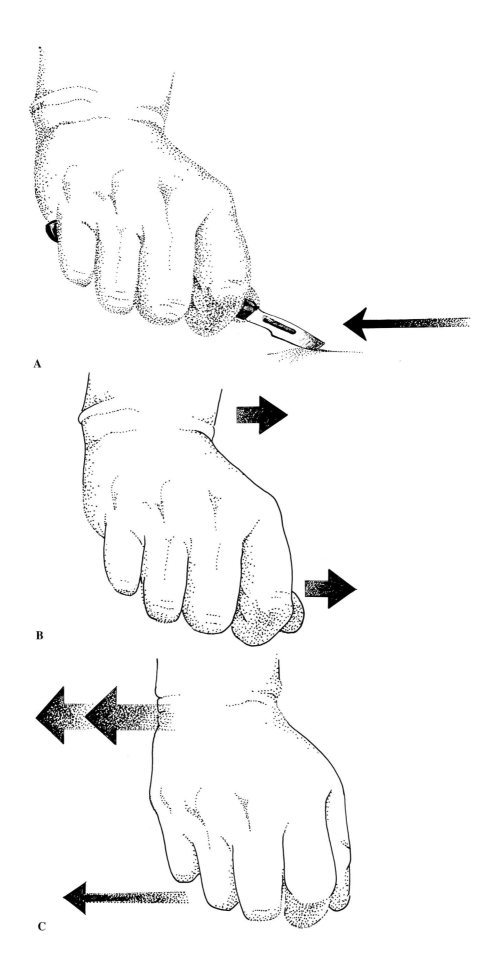

**Figure 8.10**

A

B

C

## "Suture"

The characteristic motion of sewing with a needle holder is the cocking back of the hand and wrist into a position of pronation and extension. This is followed by a flexing and supination movement that mimics driving the point of the needle through the tissues as shown in Figure 8.11A.

This motion is easily imitated and gives us the hand signal used by the surgeon when he is ready for the next suture. This pronating-supinating motion of the hand and wrist (Fig. 8.11B–C) is repeated two or three times for clarity with emphasis on the supination component.

In requesting the scissors, the surgeon finds it most convenient to signal by opening and closing the extended long and index fingers. The fingers thus simulate the blades of the scissors.

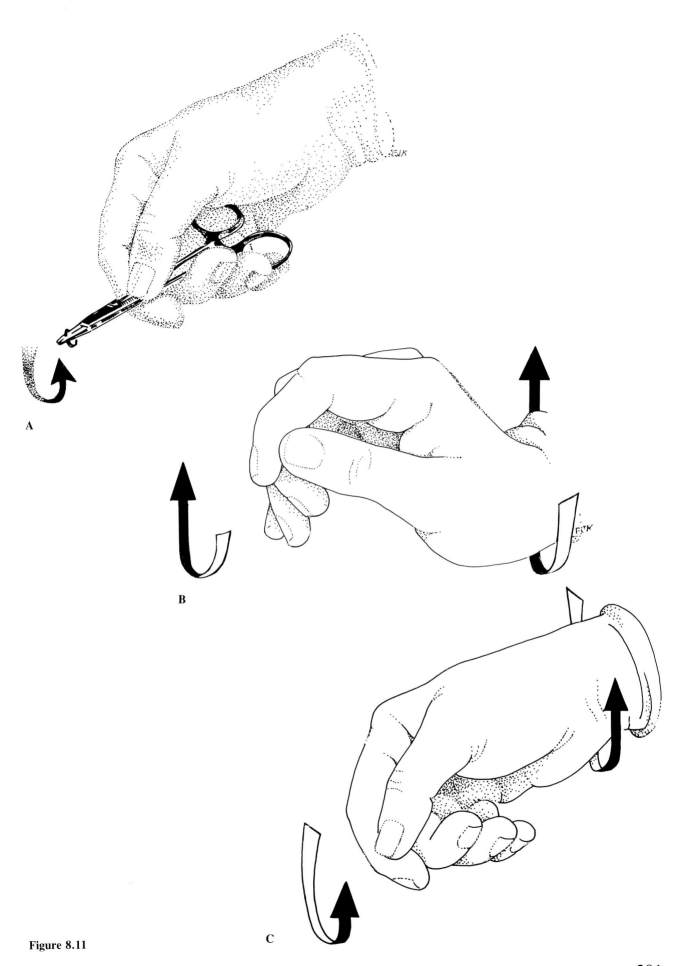

**Figure 8.11**

A

B

C

201

## "Scissors"

As noted in Figure 8.12A, the long and index fingers are not, in fact, extended when actually using the scissors. In this case, the hand signal does not duplicate the position of the hand when the instrument is held. However, the finger-snipping motions produced by the repeated spreading and closing of the index and long fingers (shown in Figure 8.12B–C) are easily understood to mean "scissors," and the signal is not likely to be confused with any other.

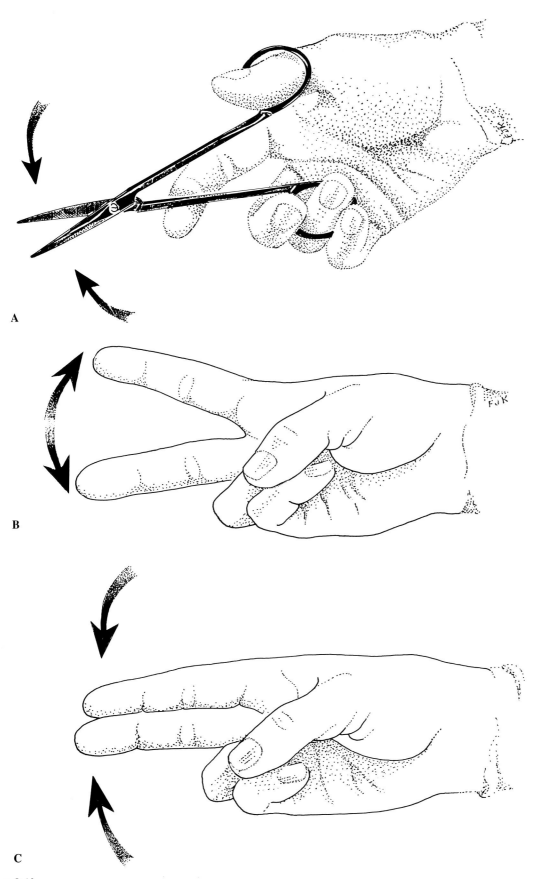

A

B

C

**Figure 8.12**

## "Skin Hook"

The use of a skin hook (or rake retractor) requires placing its prongs into the tissue as shown in Figure 8.13*A*. As in the case of the hand signal for scissors, the number of fingers flexed allows the surgeon to mimic the shape of a single-, double-, or triple-pronged hook. Thus, the hand signal (Fig. 8.13*B–C*) will show the number of prongs by the number of flexed fingers. The motion of flexing and withdrawing the wrist suggests the setting motion of the hook that fixes it in the wound margin. Note that the flexed fingers are kept separated and that the amount of flexion in the proximal and distal interphalangeal joints and in the metacarpophalangeal joints remains the same throughout the motions.

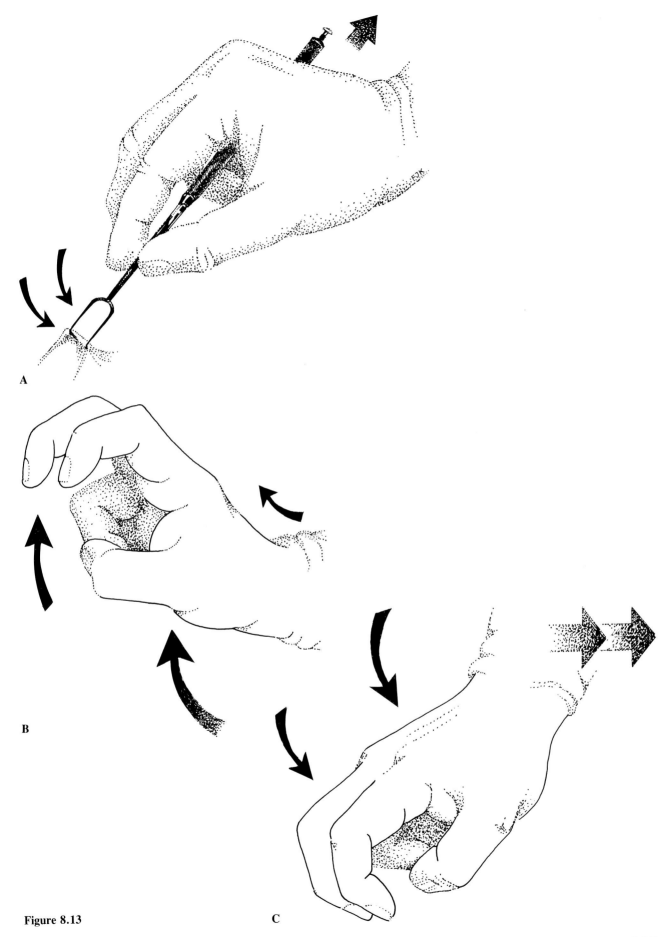

**A**

**B**

**C**

**Figure 8.13**

205

## "Syringe"

Injections with a needle and syringe produce characteristic positions and motions of the hands. In Figure 8.14A the surgeon is pushing the barrel of his syringe to inject anesthetic. Note the thumb occupies the central ring, with the index and long fingers in the two lateral rings.

This hand motion is simply reduplicated in the hand signal when the surgeon wishes to inject more local anesthetic. He uses his hand to repeat several times the motion for emptying a syringe (Fig. 8.14B–C). The thumb interphalangeal joint is kept straight during both the opening and closing motions, and the metacarpophalangeal joints of the index and long fingers are also allowed to flex only slightly.

These are only some of the commonest of the surgical hand signals. As scrub nurses work for longer periods with individual surgeons, the vocabulary of these signs will increase. At times an outstanding scrub nurse even seems to know what instrument the surgeon needs *before* he gives a hand signal. Such beautiful cooperation is indeed a joy to behold!

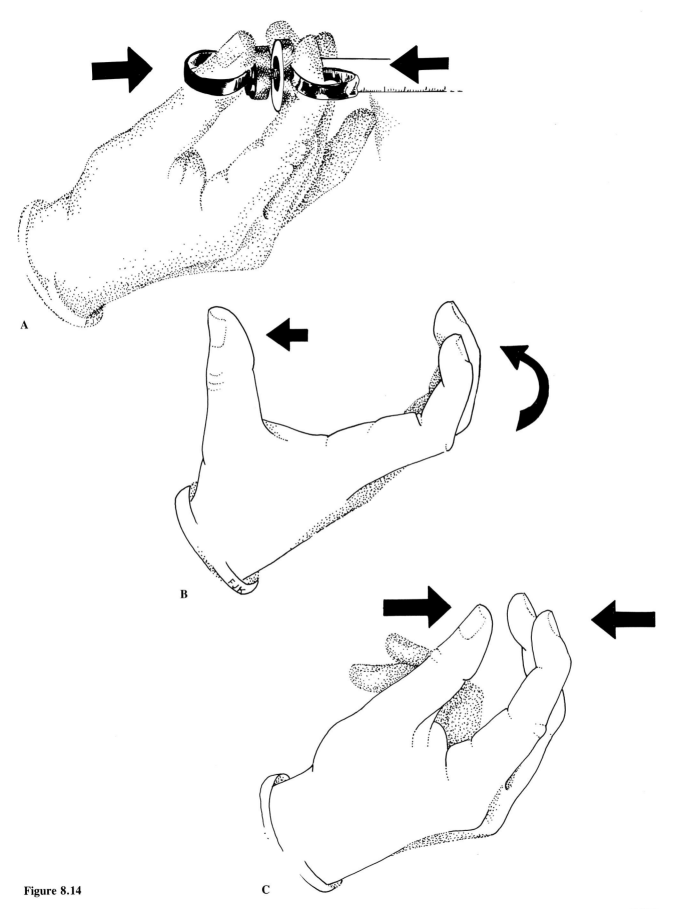

**Figure 8.14**

A

B

C

Few occupations in life cause the stress or tension of surgery, but when proper surgical judgments are made and a skilled team works efficiently to relieve a disorder, the rewards and satisfactions are enormous—not only for the patient and family, but also for the doctors and nurses on the operating team.

As technology advances in medicine, we must try to retain those arts and skills that make the application of medical science both effective and safe.

Life is short—but art is long!

*The opportunity to learn walks with any surgeon
who enters the operating room with questions on his
mind.*

Charles G. Drake quoting Wilder Penfield in his Presidential
Address at the American Surgical Association April 21, 1987

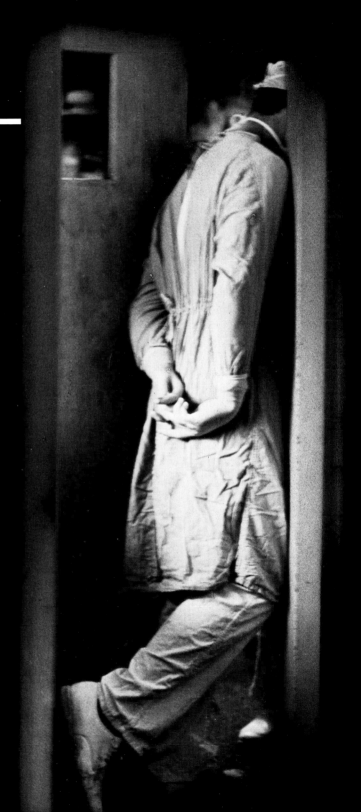

# Index

Page numbers in *italics* denote figures.

**A**

Ace bandages, 167
  cautions regarding use, 167
Adson forceps, 48, *48*, 95
Alloplastic implant materials, 180–182
  causes of postoperative infection,
      180–181
  contraindications to use, 181, *181*
  cutting and shaping with hemostatic
      (Shaw) scalpel, 68
  failures with, 181
  necessity for proper surgical technique,
      181
  uses for, 68, 181
Ambidexterity, 38
Anesthetics, local, injection techniques,
      *188,* 188–189, *190*
  angle of needle introduction, 189
  in heavily sedated patient, 189
  methods to reduce needle pain, 189
      addition of sodium bicarbonate solu-
          tion to syringe, 189
      use of fine needle, 189
  patient preparation, 189
  surgeon's demeanor, 188–189
Antibiotic solutions, 106, 159
  catheter-instilled, 159, *159*
  choice of antibiotic, 106
  irrigation of wound during surgery,
      106
  topical dressing, 159
Assistant surgeon
  anticipating need for drains and
      dressings, 153–154
  cautery technique for hemostasis,
      95–97, *96*
  cleaning and preparing operative field,
      149
  discussing postoperative management
      and dangers, 154
  education of, F1–F2
  educational opportunities during sur-
      gery, 154

method of fixing skin for incision, 3,
    5–7, *7,* 18
responsibilities during dissection, 68
responsibilities in performing pinch test
    for motor nerve identifica-
    tion, 188
responsibilities of removing blood and
    clots from wounds
  by irrigation, 105–106
  by sponging, 101
  by suction, 102
roles during surgery
  anticipating surgeon's needs
      throughout operation, 6
roles of
  asking questions, 7
  facilitating surgeon's job, 6–7
  monitoring surgical situation, 6–7
suturing and knot tying
  cutting sutures, 26–27, *27,* 35–38,
      118
    cuts "right on the knot", 37
    maintaining view of operating
        field, 36–37
    metallic sutures, 38
    method of holding scissors, *27,*
        27–28, 36, *37*
      position in palm of hand be-
          tween uses, *28,* 28–29
    moving sutures, 37–38
  hand position when passing instru-
      ments, 150, *150*
  needle fixation and presentation,
      152–153, *152–153*
  passing used needle and holder to
      nurse, 118
  receiving needle from surgeon, 118,
      *118*
  technique when assistant is tying
      knots, 118, *119–121,*
      150–151, *151*
  technique when surgeon is tying
      knots, 122, *122*

suturing responsibilities, 118–122,
    *119–122,* 148–154
wound retraction responsibilities,
    57–58

**B**

Bacitracin solution, uses of, 106, 159
Balloon tamponade, to achieve hemosta-
    sis, 100
Barton dressing, 163
Blood, removal from wounds, 100–106.
    *See also* Hemostasis
  by irrigation, 104–106, *105*
    with physiologic saline, 104–106,
        *105*
      irrigation under pressure, 105
      purposes, 104
      reduction of infection, 106
      technique, *105,* 105–106
    with topical antibiotic solutions, 106
      bacitracin, 106
  by sponging, 101, *101*
    counting and tagging sponges, 101
    technique, 101
  by suction, 102–104, *102–104*
    disadvantages, 102
    position of suction cannula, 102,
        *102*
    use during suturing, 104, *104*
    when cannula becomes blocked,
        102, *103*
Bone carpentry, 179–180, *180*
  preservation of bone circulation, 179
  special instruments used, 179
    hazards of electric or air-driven
        tools, 179
    technique of using power drill, 179,
        *180*
  surgical principles, 180
Bone wax, use in bleeding bone, 97, *97*
Brown-Adson forceps, 48, *48*
Bupivacaine, 189
  combined with epinephrine, 98

211

**C**

Casts, *162,* 162–163
    attention to detail when applying,
        162–163
    functions, 162
    proper fitting, 162–163
Catgut sutures, 76
    setting proper knot tension, 148–149
Cellulose, topical, to arrest bleeding, 98
Chemical peel techniques, 186
Clamps
    Kelly, 84, 86, 192
    mosquito, 95
    operating room hand signal for, 192,
        *193*
    Potts occlusion, 94, *94*
Cocaine solution, to achieve hemostasis,
    98
Collodion gauze patches, use after suture
        removal, *175,* 176
    application technique, 176
    skin hypersensitivity reactions, 176
Cotton sutures, 76
Cutting skin, 1–21

**D**

Dermabrasion, 186
    comparison with razabrasion, 186
    on frozen skin, 186
Dermatome, 14–16
    cautions regarding use, 15–16
    electric and air-driven models, 15, *15*
        advantages of, 15
    Padgett, 14–15
    Reece, *14,* 14–15
    technique, 14–15
    use in tropical, humid climates, 15–16
Dexon sutures, setting proper knot
        tension, 148–149
Dissection, 59–68
    assistant surgeon's role, 68
        anticipating surgeon's needs, 68
        managing hemostasis, 68
        protecting exposed tissue, 68
        repositioning of spotlights, 68
        resetting retractors as field of work
            shifts, 68
    with electrocautery, 67–68
        adjusting frequency of current, 67
        incidence of postoperative wound
            seromas, 68
    with fingertips, 61–62, *61–62*
        bidigital dissection and palpation
            technique, *61,* 61–62
        to enlarge a pocket within tissue, 62,
            *62*
    with hemostatic scalpel, 68, *68*
        use in deep tissues, 68
        use in skin, 68
    with knife, 65–66
        cautions regarding use, 65
        necessity for sharp blade, 65
        press cutting of scar under tension,
            65–66, *66*
        advantages of, 65
        with double-edged knife, 66, *67*

with Freer knife, 66, *67*
    "known-to-unknown" approach,
        66
    with olive-tip or "button-ended"
        knife, 66, *67*
    proper knife strokes, 66
    technique, 65
with laser, 67
    disadvantages, 67
with scissors, 65. *See also* Scissors
with sponges or gauze, 63–64, *63–65*
    applied by several extended fingers,
        *63,* 63–64
    use of Kuttner pledget ("peanut"),
        64, *64–65*
    wrapped around finger, 63, *63*
Dog ears, 182, *183–185*
    definition, 182
    technique for removal, 182, *183–185*
Dott-Dingman mouth gag, 50, *51*
Drains, 153, 158
    closed suction drainage, 170–171, *171*
        differences from open drainage, 170
        effect of applying suction, 171
        management of blocked catheter,
            171
        placement of drain, 171, *171*
        suturing drain to skin, 171
        use of delayed suture for later
            wound closure, 171, *171*
    combined with wet dressing for con-
        taminated wounds, 158
    how long to leave in place, 168
    management of postoperative hema-
        toma, 168, *169*
        reopening part of wound, 168, *169*
        use of grooved director, 168, *169*
    open drainage, 170, *170*
        technique of suturing drain in place,
            170, *170*
        use of delayed suture for later
            wound closure, 170, *170*
    possibility of retrograde entry of bac-
        teria, 168
    when to use, 168, 170
        reducing surgical infections, 168,
            170
Dressings, 154, 157–168
    Barton, 163
    how to apply wrapped dressings, 157
    to kill wound bacteria, 159
        use of antibiotic ointment, 159
        use of catheter to instill antibiotic
            solution, 159, *159*
    preparation of hairy areas of skin, 157
    pressure dressings, 167
        elastic (Ace bandages), 167
            cautions regarding use, 167
        nonelastic, 167
    to promote wound drainage, 158
        use of ointment-impregnated gauze,
            157–158
        beeswax base vs. petrolatum base,
            157–158
    for psychological or aesthetic needs,
        167–168

purposes, 157–168
    to reduce tissue tension on healing
        wounds, 163–167
        adhesive skin tapes, *164,* 164–165
            avoiding shear burns of skin, *164,*
                165
            for emergency treatment of lacera-
                tions, 165
            how to apply, 157
            skin hypersensitivity reactions,
                165
            use in conjunction with interrupted
                skin sutures, *164,* 164–165
        Logan bow, 165–167, *166*
            preparation for application, 165
            use in children, 167
            uses for, 165
    significance of proper application, 157
    skin protection, 157
    to splint wound, 159–163
        casts and rigid external dressings,
            *162,* 162–163
            attention to detail when applying,
                162–163
            external pin fixation, 163
            functions, 162
            proper fitting, 162–163
        to elevate a body part, 163
            overhead suspension to bedframe,
                163
            pillow technique, 163
        splinting one structure to protect
            another, 163
            fixing upper eyelid closed, 163
            intermaxillary fixation, 163
        splinting painful joints or muscles,
            163
        splinting skin grafts with tie-on
            bolus dressing, 160–161,
            *160–161*
            in children, 161
            length of time needed, 161
            purpose, 160
            technique, 161
    for wound protection, 157
        importance of fine mesh gauze, 157,
            *158*
        use of elbow splints when dressing
            children's hand wounds, 157
Dusting technique (cautery), *96,* 97

**E**

Education of surgeons, 154. *See also*
        Assistant surgeon
    handling of instruments, xix
    history, xix
    importance of hands, xx, xxi, xxiii
    importance of plastic surgery princi-
        ples, xix–xx
Electrocautery
    for dissection
        adjusting frequency of current, 68
        incidence of postoperative wound
            seromas, 68
    for hemostasis, 71, 74, 95–97, *96*
        advantages of bipolar cautery, 95

Electrocautery (*Continued*)
  cautions regarding use, 95
  direct application to vessels (dusting technique), *96,* 97
  history of use, 95
  techniques, 95–97, *96*
    necessity for dry surgical field, 95
    power setting, 95
    when to remove current, 97
    when to turn on current, 95
Embolism, deliberate, to achieve hemostasis, 98–100, *99*
  intra-arterial embolism, 98–100
    method of preventing straying emboli, *99,* 100
    problem of straying emboli, *99,* 100
    when to perform surgery after embolization, 98, 100
  intravascular balloon tamponade, 100
  when to perform embolization, 98
Epinephrine, to achieve hemostasis, 97–98
  combined with bupivacaine, 98
  dosage, 97
  injection near pedicles of flaps, 98
  in long operations, 98
  time to become effective, 97
  use with local vs. general anesthesia, 98
External pin fixation, 163

**F**
Ferris Smith knife, 11, *11*
Fingers
  importance of surgeon's hands, xix, xxi, xxiii
  use for dissecting tissues, 61–62, *61–62*
    bidigital dissection and palpation technique, *61,* 61–62
    to enlarge a pocket within tissue, 62, *62*
  use for holding tissues, 41–45, *42–44*
    necessity for moist, clean gloves, 45
    to separate adhesions, *44,* 45
    during suturing of skin incision, 41, *42–43,* 114, *114*
    Staige Davis technique of using folded sponge, 41, *42–43*
    tactile advantages, 41, 45
  use in obtaining hemostasis. *See also* Hemostasis
    bidigital compression (pinch method), *73,* 73–74
    for direct occlusion of hole in vessel, 71
    advantages over use of sponge, 71, *72*
    pressure against underlying bone, 71, *72*
Forceps, 46, *48–49,* 48–50, 182
  Adson, 48, *48,* 95
  Brown-Adson, 48, *48*
  to hold knot for tying, 148, *148*
  methods to reduce trauma with toothed forceps, *49,* 49–50

careful selection of tissue to grasp, *49,* 49–50
  gentle pressure, 49, *49*
  mouse-tooth, 48
  necessity for light springs, 48
  operating room hand signal for, 194, *195*
  smooth-jawed vs. toothed, 46, 48
    when to use smooth-jawed forceps, 48
  to stabilize tissue for suturing, *113,* 114, 116, *117*
  varieties of, 48, *48*
  Wainstock, 48, *48,* 71, *72,* 95
Free-hand technique for cutting skin grafts, 11–14
  advantages of, 14
  Ferris Smith knife, 11, *11*
  Humby knife, 13
  knife guards, 13
  preparing donor skin, 12, *12*
  surgeon's motions, 13, *13*
  use in tropical, humid climates, 14
  use of suction box, *12,* 12–13
  varying graft thickness, 13–14
Freer knife, for press cutting of scar under tension, 66, *67*
Freon, to freeze skin for dermabrasion, 186
Full-thickness skin grafts
  closure of donor site defects, *141,* 141–142
  cutting graft, *17,* 18, *19*
    determining proper depth of cut, 18
    elevation of graft, 18, *19*
    maintaining tension on skin, 18
    surgeon's motions, 18
    use of #15 blade, 18
    use of skin hooks, 18, *19*
  healing of donor site, 16
  protection of graft, 18
    defatting process, 18
    storage precautions, 18
  splinting with tie-on bolus dressing, 160–161, *160–161*
    in children, 161
    length of time needed, 161
    purpose, 160
    technique, 161
  use of patterns, *16–17,* 16–18
Furacin, 159

**G**
Gauze
  importance of fine mesh gauze for dressings, 157, *158*
  ointment-impregnated, 157–158
    beeswax base vs. petrolatum base, 157–158
    to promote wound drainage, 158
  sponge to fix moist or oily skin, 3, 5–6, *7*
  use of collodion gauze patches after suture removal, *175,* 176
Gel foam blocks, to arrest bleeding, 92, *93,* 98

Goals of surgery, xxi
Granny knot, 148
Grooved director, use of, 168, *169*

**H**
Halsted roll, 117, 138
Hand signals in operating room, 191–203, *193, 195–198, 200–202*
  importance of maintaining quiet operating room, 191
  responsibilities of scrub nurse, 192, 203
  signal for clamp, 192, *193*
  signal for forceps, 194, *195*
  signal for large-bladed scalpel, 199, *199*
  signal for scissors, 202, *203*
  signal for skin hook (rake retractor), 204, *205*
  signal for small-bladed scalpel, 196, *197*
  signal for suture, 200, *201*
  signal for syringe, 206, *207*
Hematoma, postoperative management, 168
  reopening part of wound, 168, *169*
  use of grooved director, 168, *169*
Hemostasis, 69–100
  by cautery, 95–97, *96*
    advantages of bipolar cautery, 95
    cautions regarding use, 95
    direct application to vessels (dusting technique), *96,* 97
    history of use, 95
    necessity for dry surgical field, 95
    techniques, 95–97, *96*
    power setting, 95
    when to remove current, 97
    when to turn on current, 95
  with drugs, 97–98
    controlled systemic hypotension, 98
      advantages of, 98
    topical clotting agents, 98
      length of application, 98
      removal of, 98
    vasoconstrictors, 97–98
      cocaine solution, 98
      dosage, 97
      injection near pedicles of flaps, 98
      in long operations, 98
      time to become effective, 97
      use with local vs. general anesthesia, 98
  historical methods of arresting bleeding, 71
  by intravascular occlusion of regional vessels, 98–100, *99*
    intra-arterial embolism, 98–100, *99*
      method of preventing straying emboli, *99,* 100
      problem of straying emboli, *99,* 100
      when to perform surgery after embolization, 98, 100

Hemostasis (*Continued*)
    intravascular balloon tamponade,
        100
        when to perform embolization, 98
    by ligatures and metal clips, 76–91
        pros and cons of metal clips, *90,*
            *90–91*
        tying techniques. *See also* Knots
            instrument tie-in-a-hole, 86–90,
                *87–90*
            tie-on-a-clamp, 84–86, *84–86*
            two-handed tie, 76–82, *78–83*
        types of ligatures, 76
            absorbable vs. nonabsorbable, 76
            flexible vs. rigid, 76
            natural materials vs. synthetics, 76
            pros and cons of nylon, 76
            pros and cons of silk, 76
        where to apply ligatures, 76
    by pressure, 71–76
        bidigital compression (pinch
            method), *73,* 73–74
            advantage of hemostasis early in
                operation, 74
            assistant's hand position, 73, *73*
        direct occlusion of hole in vessel by
            fingertip, 71
            advantages over use of sponge,
                71, *72*
        packing, 75–76
            control of deep bleeding, 76
            cool vs. warm saline for moisten-
                ing packs, 75
            long-term packing, 76
            moist vs. dry packs, 75
        pressure against underlying bone,
            71, *72*
        serial release of finger pressure to
            identify bleeders, 71
        pressure with knife or instrument tip,
            74, *74*
        sponge and sponge stick pressure,
            *75,* 75–76
    by suture ligatures, 91–94, *91–94*
        direct suture of vessel walls, 94, *94*
        patch repair of vessel walls, 94, *94*
        placing sutures through vessels, *91,*
            91–92
            technique, 91
            use in conjunction with ties, 91
            use of two-handed tie, 92
            where to suture, 91
        suture of buried bleeders, 92, *92–93*
        temporary suture tourniquet of ves-
            sels in continuity, 92, *93*
            indications for, 92
            use of slip knot, 92, *93*
    by twist occlusion, 76, *77*
        contraindications to use, 76
        French twist method, 76
    use of Shaw scalpel, 68, *68*
    by vessel plugging in bleeding bone,
        97, *97*
        use of bone wax, 97, *97*
Hilton's maneuver, use of scissors,
    32–34, *33–34*

Humby knife, 13
Hypotension, controlled systemic, to
    achieve hemostasis, 98
    advantages of, 98

**I**
Injection techniques for local anesthetics,
    *188,* 188–189, *190*
    angle of needle introduction, 189
    in heavily sedated patient, 189
    methods to reduce needle pain, 189
        addition of sodium bicarbonate solu-
            tion to syringe, 189
        use of fine needle, 189
    patient preparation, 189
    surgeon's demeanor, 188–189
Irrigation, to remove blood and clots
        from wounds, 104–106, *105*
    with physiologic saline, 104–106, *105*
        irrigation under pressure, 105
        purposes, 104
        reduction of infection, 106
        technique, 105–106
    with topical antibiotic solutions, 106
        bacitracin, 106

**J**
Jamieson scissors, 26, *26,* 30

**K**
Keith needle, 109
Kelly clamp, 84, 86, 192
Knife. *See* Scalpel
Knife guards, use of, 13
Knots. *See also* Suturing
    deep placement of knots for subcuticu-
        lar sutures, 122–123, *123*
    granny, 148
    requirements when tying, 78, 104
    for running intradermal pull-out su-
        tures, 126
    slip knot, for temporary suture tourni-
        quet of vessels in continuity,
        92, *93*
    square, 79–82, *79–83,* 118, *121,* 128
    surgeon's, 146, 148
    suture tension
        judging tension, 143, *143*
        setting proper tension, 144–149
            with absorbable sutures, 148–149
            with metallic sutures, 149, *149*
            with silk sutures, 144–148,
                *144–148*
            with synthetic suture materials,
                148, *148*
    tying techniques
        instrument tie-in-a-hole, 86–90,
            *87–90*
        first throw (two-handed tie), 86,
            89
        second throw (two-handed tie),
            89–90, *89–90*
        one-handed knot tying, 146, *147*

tie-on-a-clamp, 84–86, *84–86*
    when point of clamp holding
        bleeder faces away from sur-
        geon, 86, *86*
two-handed tie, 76–82, *78–83,* 145,
    149
    avoiding obstruction of assistant's
        view, 78, *78,* 81
    for placing sutures through ves-
        sels, 92
    the first throw, 79–81, *79–81*
    the second throw, 82, *82–83*
use of needle holder when tying, 109,
    118–122, *119–122,* 145, 149
technique when assistant is tying,
    118, *119–121,* 150–151, *151*
technique when surgeon is tying,
    122, *122*
Kocher clamp, use as retractor on ne-
    crotic tissue, 56, *56*
Kuttner pledget ("peanut"), use for dis-
    section, 64, *64–65*

**L**
Laser, use for dissection, 67
Lashal scissors, for suture removal, *173,*
    174
Left-handed surgeon, 191
    use of right- vs. left-handed scissors,
        31–32
Lidocaine, 189
Ligatures
    suture ligatures, 91–94, *91–94. See
        also* Suturing
    tying techniques. *See also* Knots
        instrument tie-in-a-hole, 86–90,
            *87–90*
        one-handed tie, 146, *147*
        tie-on-a-clamp, 84–86, *84–86*
        two-handed tie, 76–82, *78–83*
    types of, 76
        absorbable vs. nonabsorbable, 76
        flexible vs. rigid, 76
        natural materials vs. synthetics, 76
        pros and cons of nylon, 76
        pros and cons of silk, 76
    where to apply, 76
Logan bow, 165–167, *166*
    preparation for application, 165
    use in children, 167
    uses for, 165

**M**
Marcaine. *See* Bupivacaine
Mayo scissors, 26
Metal clips, *90,* 90–91
    pros and cons, *90,* 90–91
    radiopacity, 91
    uses of, 90
Metallic sutures, 38
    setting proper knot tension, 149, *149*
Metzenbaum scissors, 20, 26, *26,* 30, 36

**N**

Needle fixation and presentation technique, 152–153, *152–153*

Needle holder, 112–114, *112–115*
designating choice of needle and suture, 112, 114
how to receive from nurse, 112, *112*
position of suture material, 112, *112*
use when tying sutures, 109, 118–122, *119–122*, 145, 149
selecting proper needle holder, 109
windowed, for suturing in narrow deep spaces, 137, *137*

Needles
hand- vs. machine-sharpened, 109
handheld needles, 109, *110*
use of straight cutting needle, 109, *110*
hand-threaded vs. swaged-on sutures, 109
increasing curve of, to suture in narrow deep spaces, 137, *137*
Keith, 109
selecting according to task, 109

Neomycin, 159

Novafil sutures, 126

Nylon sutures, 76, 109, 125–126, 141, 174
setting proper knot tension, 148, *148*

**O**

Operating table, correct height, 4–5, *5*
distance between operative field and eyes, 4
functional position of wrist, 4–5, *5*
for surgery on depressed body surface or body cavity, 5

**P**

Packing, to achieve hemostasis, 75–76
control of deep bleeding, 76
cool vs. warm saline for moistening, 75
long-term packing, 76
moist vs. dry packs, 75
"Peanut" dissection, 64, *64–65*
Phenolic acid, use for chemical peel, 186
Physiologic saline, to irrigate wounds, 104–106, *105*
Pinch method, of obtaining hemostasis, *73*, 73–74. *See also* Hemostasis
Pinch test, for motor nerve identification, 186, 188
comparison with nerve stimulators, 186, 188
reliability, 188
technique, 188
Plaster of Paris casts, 162–163
Postoperative wound hematoma, 168, *169*
Potts occlusion clamp, 94, *94*
Pressure dressings, 167
elastic, 167
nonelastic, 167

Prolene sutures, 126, 174
setting proper knot tension, 148, *148*

**R**

Razabrasion, 11, 186, *187*
advantages of, 186
comparison to dermabrasion, 186
how to hold blade, *10, 187*
indications for, 11
skin surfaces where contraindicated, 11
type of razor blade used, *10, 11*, 186
Retractors, 50–58, *51–58*
avoiding tissue injury with, 45, 50
differences between types of retractors, 52
muscle necrosis, 52, *53*
protection of wound margins, *44, 45*, 52
surgeon's breath-holding technique, 52
handheld, 50, 52, *53*
advantages, 50, 52
importance of adequate incision, 50
moving wound principle to increase exposure, 57–58, *57–58*
self-retaining, 50, *51–52*
disadvantages of, 50
Dott-Dingman mouth gag, 50, *51*
spring-loaded vs. locking, 50
sutures, 54–55, *54–55*
to bring inaccessible tissue into view, 55, *55*
importance of holding clamps on suture ends, 54
tissue-crushing instruments, 56, *56*
indications for use, 56
Kocher clamp, 56, *56*
types of, 50–55

**S**

Scalpel
for dissection, 65–66
cautions regarding use, 65
necessity for sharp blade, 65
press cutting of scar under tension, 65–66, *66*
advantages, 65
with double-edged knife, 66, *67*
with Freer knife, 66, *67*
"known-to-unknown" approach, 66
with olive-tip or "button-ended" knife, 66, *67*
proper knife strokes, 66
technique, 65
hemostatic, 68, *68*
methods of holding, 5–6
power grip, 3, *4*, 5
when to use, 5
precision grip, 5–6, *7*
eliminating hand tremor, 6
when to use, 5–6
for occluding open ends of transected blood vessels, 74, *74*

operating room hand signal for
large-bladed knife, 194, *197*
small-bladed knife, 194, *196*
pressure with knife to arrest bleeding, 74, *74*
removing sutures with #11 blade, 172, *172*
Shaw, 68, *68*
special blades, 8–9
#12, 9, *9*
#11 blade, 8–9, *8–9*
olive-tip or "button-ended", 66, *67*
double-edged, 66, *67*
Freer, 66, *67*
right-angled blades, 9, *9*
Scissors, 23–38
for cutting skin, 20
avoiding buttonholing skin, 18, 38
knife-then-scissors technique, 20, *21*
for cutting sutures, 26–27, *27*, 35–38
buried sutures, 35–36
metallic sutures, 38
method of holding scissors, 27–28, *28, 36, 37*
position in palm of hand between uses, *28*, 28–29
moving sutures, 37–38
proper length of suture ends, 35, *35*
skin sutures, 35
technique, 36–37
cuts "right on the knot", 37
how to hold, *27*, 27–30
fixation and control grips, *27*, 27–28
increasing tactile control, 29–30, *29–30*
to identify depth of dissection, 30
stripping technique, 30, *31*
when deep surface of skin is scarred, 30, *30*
position in palm of hand between uses, *28*, 28–29
Jamieson, 26, *26*, 30
Lashal, for suture removal, *173*, 174
Mayo, 26
mechanics of, 31–32
how the handle produces shear forces, 31–32
"tips-toward-wrist" grip, 32, *32*
indications for, 32
unusual grips, 32
left-handed scissors, 31–32
right-handed scissors, 31–32
Metzenbaum, 20, 26, *26*, 30, 36
operating room hand signal for, 194, 199, *200*
surgical functions of, 32, 34, 65
for undermining skin, *30*, 65
importance of counter traction on skin edge, 30
palpation of skin flap thickness with left hand, *30*, 30
use in combination with other instruments, 38
ambidexterity, 38
bimanual techniques, 38

Scissors (*Continued*)
    use in Hilton's maneuver, 32–34,
        *33–34*
    varieties of, 25–27
        curved vs. straight blades, 26
        differences among, 25
        handle length, 25
        sharpness of scissor tips, *25,* 25–26
        special designs, 27
Scope of book, xiii
    audience, xi, xx
    criteria for including techniques, xiii
    purposes, xx, xxi
Shaw scalpel, 68, *68*
Silk sutures, 76, 109, 126
    setting proper knot tension, 144–148,
        *144–148*
Skin
    anatomy, 3
    cutting tangentially, 9–20
        full-thickness skin grafts, 16–20. *See
            also* Full-thickness skin grafts
        indications for, 9
        partial (split-thickness) skin sections,
            9–16. *See also* split-thickness
            skin grafts
    cutting with scissors, 20
        avoiding buttonholing, 18, 38
        knife-then-scissors technique, 20, *21*
    holding or fixing during incision, 3
        by assistant, 3, 5, *7*
        importance of maintaining skin ten-
            sion, 3, 5–6
        for long incisions, 3, *4,* 5
        method of gripping scalpel, 3, *4,* 5
        by surgeon's nondominant hand, 3,
            *4, 6, 7*
        use of sponges to fix moist or oily
            skin, 3, 5–6, *7*
    importance of proper handling, xx, xxi
    instruments for holding, 39–58. *See
        also* specific instruments
        fingers, 41–45, *42–44*
        forceps, 46, *48–49,* 48–50
        retractors, 50–58, *51–58*
        skin hooks, 45–46, *45–47*
    suturing, 116–122. *See also* Suturing
        inserting needle, 116, *116*
            surgeon's hand position, 116, *116*
        obtaining ideal skin approximation,
            116, *116–117*
            everting skin edges with forceps
                or skin hook, 116
            second side of incision, 116, *117*
            vertical lifting of suture line
                (Halsted roll), 116, *116*
        with running cuticular suture,
            128–133
            advantages and disadvantages, 128
            technique of suture placement,
                128–133, *129–132*
        with running intradermal pull-out su-
            ture, 126–128
            advantages, 126
            technique of suture placement,
                126–128, *127*

use of fingers to hold tissue, 41,
    *42–43*
Skin grafts
    affixing to wound margins with run-
        ning cuticular sutures, 133,
        *133*
    cutting grafts, 9–18
        with dermatomes, *14–15,* 14–16
        free-hand knife method, *11–13,*
            11–14
        with razor blade, *10,* 11, 186, *187*
        with scalpel, *17,* 18, *19*
    dressings
        open, 9
        tie-on bolus, 160–161, *160–161*
    full-thickness. *See* Full-thickness skin
        grafts
    split-thickness. *See* Split-thickness skin
        grafts
    suturing, 109, *110–111*
Skin hooks, 45–46, *45–47*
    contraindications to use, 46
    design requirements, 45
    method of setting tips in tissue, 46, *47*
    operating room hand signal for, 199,
        *201*
    uses of, 18, *19,* 30, *61,* 62, 182, *183*
        to stabilize tissue for suturing, *113,*
            114, 116, *124–125,*
            124–126, *127,* 130, *131,*
            138, *139,* 146, *147*
    varieties of, 46, *46*
Sodium bicarbonate, use when injecting
    local anesthetics, 189
Splints. *See* Dressings
Split-thickness skin grafts, 9–16
    healing of donor site, 9
    large tangential cuts (split-thickness
        grafts), 11–16
        dermatomes, 14–16
            cautions regarding use, 15–16
            electric and air-driven models, 15,
                *15*
                advantages of, 15
            Padgett dermatome, 14–15
            Reece dermatome, *14,* 14–15
            technique, 14–15
            use in tropical, humid climates,
                15–16
        free-hand knife method, 11–14
            advantages of, 14
            Ferris Smith knife, 11, *11*
            Humby knife, 13
            knife guards, 13
            preparing donor skin, 12, *12*
            surgeon's motions, 13, *13*
            use in tropical, humid climates,
                14
            use of suction box, *12,* 12–13
            varying graft thickness, 13–14
        indications for, 11
    small tangential cuts of split-thickness
        skin, 11
        technique of razabrasion, *10,* 11,
            186, *187*
            advantages of, 186

comparison to dermabrasion, 186
how to hold blade, *10, 187*
indications for, 11
skin surfaces where contraindi-
    cated, 11
type of razor blade, *10,* 11, 186
suturing methods, 109, *110–111*
    pie-crust technique, 109, *111*
type of knife blade required, 9
Sponges
    to remove blood and clots from
        wounds, 101, *101*
        counting and tagging sponges, 101
        technique, 101
    to stabilize tissue for suturing, 114,
        *115*
    use in arresting bleeding by tamponade
        adherence of fresh thrombi to
            sponge, 71, *72*
        sponge and sponge stick pressure,
            *75,* 75–76
    use in arresting bleeding by tampon-
        ade, 75, *75*
Square knots. *See* Knots
Steel sutures, 38
    setting proper knot tension, 149, *149*
Steri-strips, 141, 176
Suction, to remove blood and clots from
    wound, 102–104, *102–104*
    disadvantages, 102
    position of suction cannula, 102, *102*
    use when suturing, 104, *104*
    when cannula becomes blocked, 102,
        *103*
Suction box, use when obtaining split-
    thickness skin grafts, *12,*
    12–13
Suction drainage, 170–171, *170–171. See
    also* Drains
Surgeon's knot, 146, 148
Surgical technique, importance of teach-
    ing, xix–xxi, xxiii
Suture ligatures, 91–94, *91–94*
    direct suture of vessel walls, 94, *94*
    patch repair of vessel walls, 94, *94*
    placing sutures through vessels, *91,*
        91–92
        technique, 91, *91*
        use in conjunction with ties, 91
        use of two-handed tie technique, 92
        where to apply suture, 91
    suture of buried bleeders, 92, *92–93*
    temporary suture tourniquet of vessels
        in continuity, 92, *93*
        indications for, 92
        use of slip knot, 92, *93*
Suture removal, 171–176
    buried running sutures, 174
        method for extracting a "hung-up"
            running suture, 174, *175*
    interrupted sutures, *172,* 172–174
    nonburied running sutures, 174
    running buried intradermal pull-out su-
        ture, 126
    skin fixation to replace sutures,
        175–176

Suture removal (*Continued*)
  with adhesive skin tapes, 175
  with collodion gauze patches, *175,*
      176
    application technique, 176
    skin hypersensitivity reactions, 176
  timing of, 174
    effects of leaving sutures in too
        long, 174
    measures taken during surgery to al-
        low early suture removal,
        174
  use of special instruments: Lashal scis-
      sors, *173,* 174
Suturing, 107–154
  assistant surgeon's responsibilities,
      118–122, *119–122,* 148–154.
      *See also* Assistant surgeon
  anticipating need for drains and
      dressings, 153–154
  cleaning and preparing operative
      field, 149
  discussing postoperative management
      and dangers, 154
  educational opportunities during sur-
      gery, 154
  hand position when passing instru-
      ments, 150, *150*
  needle fixation and presentation,
      152–153, *152–153*
  passing used needle and holder to
      nurse, 118
  receiving needle from surgeon, 118,
      *118*
  technique when assistant is tying
      knots, 118, *119–121,*
      150–151, *151*
  technique when surgeon is tying
      knots, 122, *122*
  cutting sutures, 118
    buried sutures, 35–36
      absorbable, 35–36
      nonabsorbable, 35–36
    cuts "right on the knot", 37
    metallic sutures, 38
    moving sutures, 37–38
    proper length of suture ends, 35, *35*
    scissors for, 26–27
    skin sutures, 35
    technique, 26–27, *27,* 35–38, *37*
  how to suture drains in place
    closed suction drains, 171, *171*
    open drains, 170, *170*
    use of delayed suture for later
        wound closure, 170–171,
        *170–171*
  mattress sutures, 134–135
    advantages of, 134
    disadvantages, 134–135
    horizontal, *134,* 134–135
    indications for, 134
    vertical, 134, *134*
  needle choice for suturing, 109
    handheld needles, 109, *110*
      use of straight cutting needle,
          109, *110*

ideal suture of future, 109
selecting according to task, 109
operating room hand signal for suture,
    194, *198*
removing dog ears, 182, *183–185*
retention ("stay") sutures, 135, *136*
  dangers of, 135
  indications for, 135
  technical precautions, 135
    method of tying, 135
    type of needle required, 135
running cuticular suture, 128–133
  advantages and disadvantages of,
      128
  to affix skin graft to wound margins,
      133, *133*
  technique of suture placement,
      128–133, *129–132*
    with assistant, 130
    choosing proper end of incision to
        begin, 128, *129–130,* 130
    with no assistant, 130, *131–132,*
        133
running intradermal pull-out suture,
    126–128
  advantages of, 126
  requirements of suture material, 126
  technique of suture placement,
      126–128, *127*
  where to use, 126
of skin, 116–122
  inserting needle, 116, *116*
    surgeon's hand position, 116, *116*
  obtaining ideal skin approximation,
      116, *116–117*
    everting skin edges with forceps
        or skin hook, 116
    second side of incision, 116, *117*
    vertical lifting of suture line
        (Halsted roll), 116, *116*
  with running cuticular suture,
      128–133
  with running intradermal pull-out su-
      ture, 126–128, *127*
  use of fingers to hold tissue, 41,
      *42–43*
    Staige Davis technique of using
        folded sponge, 41, *42–43*
of skin grafts, 109, *110–111*
  pie-crust technique, 109, *111*
special techniques, 137–141
  closure of skin defect or donor site
      with local tissues, 140–141,
      *141*
    circular defect, 141, *141*
    elliptical defect, 141, *141*
  suturing by bisection, 140, *140*
  suturing in narrow deep spaces, 137,
      *137*
    increasing curve of needle, 137,
        *137*
    use of windowed needle holder,
        137, *137*
  suturing with advancement and sew-
      ing around curves, 138,
      *138–139*

decreasing tension on sutures in
    flap tip, 138
occurrence of trap-door deformi-
    ties, 138
repositioning skin flap, 138,
    *138–139*
stabilizing tissue for suturing,
    *113–115,* 114
  with finger, 114, *114*
  with folded sponge, 114, *115*
  with forceps, *113,* 114
  with skin hook, *113,* 114, 116,
      *124–125,* 124–126, *127,*
      130, *131,* 138, *139,* 146,
      *147*
subcuticular sutures, 122–125
  contraindications to use, 122
  indications for, 122
  long-term fate of subcuticular nylon,
      125
    correct placement of sutures, 125
  placing knots deep, 122–123, *123*
  placing to cause minimal trauma,
      124–125, *124–125*
    technique, 124–125
    use of skin hook, 124–125,
        *124–125*
  problems in placing, *123,* 124
tension on sutures, 142–149
  effects of too-loose sutures, 142
  effects of too-tight sutures, 142–143
  history, 142, *142*
  judging tension, 143, *143*
  setting proper tension, 144–149
    with absorbable sutures, 148–149
    with silk sutures, 144–148,
        *144–148*
      with assistant holding first loop
          of knot, 148, *148*
      placement of knot, 145
      tying under tension, 146, *147*
      use of surgeon's knot, 146
    with synthetic suture materials,
        148, *148*
tying sutures. *See* Knots
use of needle holder, 112–114,
    *112–115*
  designating choice of needle and su-
      ture size, 112, 114
  how to receive from nurse, 112, *112*
  position of suture material, 112, *112*
  when tying knots, 109, 118–122,
      *119–122*
    advantages of, 118
    technique when assistant is tying,
        118, *119–121*
    technique when surgeon is tying,
        122, *122*
using sutures as retractors, 54–55,
    *54–55*
  to bring inaccessible tissue into
      view, 55, *55*
  importance of holding clamps on su-
      ture ends, 54
Syringe, operating room hand signal for,
    199, *202*

**T**
Tape, adhesive skin, *164,* 164–165
  avoiding shear burns of skin, *164,* 165
  for emergency treatment of lacerations, 165
  how to apply, 157
  to reduce tissue tension after sutures are removed, 175
  skin hypersensitivity reactions, 165
  use in conjunction with interrupted skin sutures, *164,* 164–165
Teeth, intermaxillary fixation, 163
Thrombin solution, to arrest bleeding, 98
Ties. *See* Knots; Ligatures
Trap-door deformity, occurring in curved skin incisions, 138

Trichloracetic acid, use for chemical peel, 186
Twist-occlusion technique for hemostasis, 76, *77*

**V**
Vasoconstrictor drugs, to achieve hemostasis, 97–98
  cocaine solution, 98
  combined with bupivacaine, 98
  dosage, 97
  epinephrine, 97–98
  injection near pedicles of flaps, 98
  in long operations, 98
  time to become effective, 97

use with local vs. general anesthesia, 98
Vicryl sutures, setting proper knot tension, 148–149

**W**
Wainstock forceps, 48, *48,* 71, *72,* 95
Wire cutters, for cutting metallic sutures, 38
Wound protection. *See* Dressings
Wrapped dressings, 157

**X**
Xeroform gauze, 157